Road Accident Statistics English Regions 1992

October 1993
London: HMSO

Prepared for publication by STD5 branch
Directorate of Statistics
Department of Transport

Richard Ackroyd
Paul O'Connor
Yuk-Shu Ho
Richard Paddock

GOVERNMENT STATISTICAL SERVICE

A service of statistical information and advice is provided to the government by specialist staff employed in the statistics divisions of individual Departments. Statistics are made generally available through their publications and further information and advice on them can be obtained from the Departments concerned.

Enquiries about the contents of this publication should be made to:

Directorate of Statistics
Department of Transport
Room B648
Romney House
43 Marsham Street
London SW1P 3PY

Telephone 071 276 8785

Data Service

Copies of the main tables in this publication can be supplied on a computer diskette by the Department of Transport (at a cost of £40). Further tabulations of road accident statistics are also available from the Department, subject to confidentiality rules. The charges vary with the complexity of the analysis (minimum £40) and the availability of these services depends upon the resources within the Department. Enquiries should be addressed in writing to Mr P S O'Connor at the above address

Contents

Symbols and Conventions

Rounding of Figures

In tables where figures have been rounded there may be an apparent slight discrepancy between the sum of the constituent items and the independently rounded total.

Symbols

The following symbols have been used throughout:

'-' = nil or negligible (less than half the final digit shown)

'..' = not available

Conversion Factor

1 kilometre = 0.6214 mile

Preface

This is the 1992 edition of Road Accident Statistics English Regions (RASER), a publication which gives statistics of road accidents on a local basis for England. RASER concentrates on accidents as being incidents which may reflect a need for local action and is intended to be of most benefit to traffic engineers, planners and administrators in local government and the Department of Transport (DOT) regional offices. For this reason, most of the data in the book are compiled according to the county groupings covered by these offices (which are shown on the map on the adjoining page).

RASER is confined to background national statistics, so it should be regarded as a supplement to 'Road Accidents Great Britain 1992 - The Casualty Report' (RAGB), which is the main publication on road accident statistics in Great Britain. RAGB is available from HMSO bookshops, price £10.95.

The current system of collecting road accident statistics was set up in 1968, and is for the benefit and use of local authorities, the police and central government. Each year, about 250,000 STATS19 road accident report forms (an example of which can be found on pages 45 to 47) are completed by police officers of the 51 police forces in Great Britain. These forms record data about accidents on the public highway which involved personal injury or death. These data are transferred onto magnetic tape or computer diskette and are sent to DOT where they are incorporated into an annual data file.

The principal purpose in collecting and publishing statistics of road accidents is to provide background information for both central government and local authorities on the roads, road users, places, times of day, weather conditions, where road accidents happen etc, and against which various remedial measures can be considered. Road accident statistics are used to provide both a local and a national perspective for particular road safety problems or particular suggested remedies. A continuous flow of information - such as the time series tables in this book - means that trends of accidents and casualties can be examined and used to change the direction of policies when necessary.

The report also includes data from Northern Ireland. These data, where available, are included with each table along with data for Scotland and Wales. *More detailed statistics for Scotland and Wales are available from the Scottish and Welsh Offices - please refer to the inside rear cover for more details.*

Several of the tables contain averages of 1981-85 data. These represent the base figures which the Secretary of State for Transport used to set the target of reducing the number of road casualties by one third by the year 2000. It should also be noted that main Tables 1 and 6 which give casualty totals by severity for the years covering 1981 to 1985 have been extended to show revised estimates for London for this period. At the beginning of September 1984 the Metropolitan police implemented improved procedures for allocating the level of severity to accidents and casualties. The change is thought to have had no effect on overall casualty numbers, but in the period between 1981 and the date of the change it is estimated that there were 4,725 casualties whose injuries were originally judged to be slight but would have been judged serious under the later procedures. However, this is an overall estimate and it is not possible to present similar revised estimates of accidents by road type and other detailed characteristics.

DOT is generally prepared to sell tabulations of road accident data. The cost of data varies with the complexity of each request, but averages about £40 per year of data. Further information can be obtained from: - *Mr Paul O'Connor, Department of Transport, Room B648, Romney House, 43 Marsham Street, London SW1P 3PY, Telephone 071-276-8785.*

DEPARTMENT OF TRANSPORT REGIONAL ORGANISATION

AS AT NOVEMBER 1991

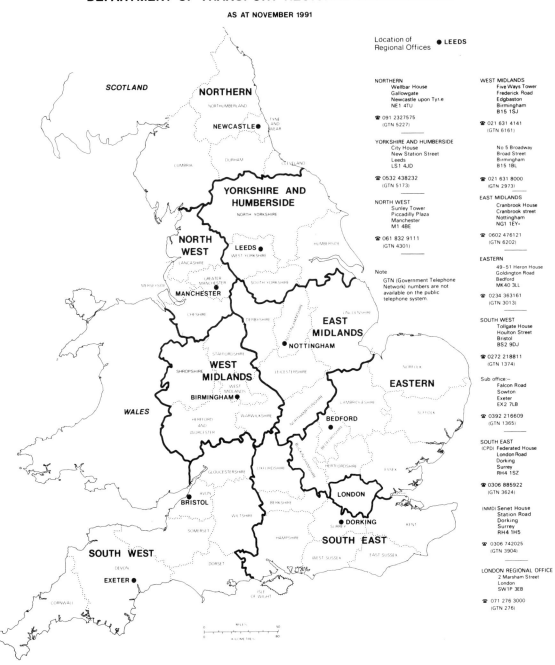

Location of Regional Offices ● LEEDS

NORTHERN
Wellbar House
Gallowgate
Newcastle upon Tyne
NE1 4TU

☎ 091 2327575
(GTN 5227)

YORKSHIRE AND HUMBERSIDE
City House
New Station Street
Leeds
LS1 4JD

☎ 0532 438232
(GTN 5173)

NORTH WEST
Sunley Tower
Piccadilly Plaza
Manchester
M1 4BE

☎ 061 832 9111
(GTN 4301)

Note

GTN (Government Telephone Network) numbers are not available on the public telephone system.

WEST MIDLANDS
Five Ways Tower
Frederick Road
Edgbaston
Birmingham
B15 1SJ

☎ 021 631 4141
(GTN 6161)

No 5 Broadway
Broad Street
Birmingham
B15 1BL

☎ 021 631 8000
(GTN 2973)

EAST MIDLANDS
Cranbrook House
Cranbrook street
Nottingham
NG1 1EY

☎ 0602 476121
(GTN 6202)

EASTERN
49-51 Heron House
Goldington Road
Bedford
MK40 3LL

☎ 0234 363161
(GTN 3013)

SOUTH WEST
Tollgate House
Houlton Street
Bristol
BS2 9DJ

☎ 0272 218811
(GTN 1374)

Sub office:-
Falcon Road
Sowton
Exeter
EX2 7LB

☎ 0392 216609
(GTN 1365)

SOUTH EAST
(CPD) Federated House
London Road
Dorking
Surrey
RH4 1SZ

☎ 0306 885922
(GTN 3624)

(NMD) Senet House
Station Road
Dorking
Surrey
RH4 1HS

☎ 0306 742025
(GTN 3904)

LONDON REGIONAL OFFICE
2 Marsham Street
London
SW1P 3EB

☎ 071 276 3000
(GTN 276)

Further copies of this map may be obtained from:
HGU Drawing Office
P2/019, 2 Marsham St.

Department of Transport
HGU Drawing Office 91 198

1. Commentary on tables and charts

Richard Ackroyd

1.1 Introduction

This section gives a review of the main body of tables included in this report. As noted in the introduction, the data in most of the tables are disaggregated either by county or Department of Transport (DOT) region and Northern Ireland data have been included within certain tables. Tables where Northern Ireland data are not available, and thus where no United Kingdom total can be given, have been individually annotated.

From 1 April 1991, responsibility for the county of Cumbria transferred from the North West region of the DOT organisation to the Northern region. The DOT accident database was amended with effect from 1 January 1992 and as a consequence the numbers and rates for 1992 as shown in this report have been based on the new organisation, but for the years up to and including 1991 the old definition has been used.

In order to provide consistent time series, the casualty data for the Northern and North West regions in Table 1 (page 21) have been calculated throughout according to the new definitions and these times series are also shown in the table below. The data for previous years in these two regions in Table 14 have also been similarly revised. However, the change in definitions means that in the remaining tables the 1992 data for these regions are not consistent with data for previous years.

Casualties: Northern and North West regions by severity: 1981-1985 average, 1986-1992

	1981–5 Average	1986	1987	1988	1989	1990	1991	1992
Northern[1]								
Killed	282	261	294	280	270	334	287	225
Killed or seriously injured	3,466	3,158	2,916	2,947	2,962	3,050	2,651	2,475
All Casualties	13,913	13,783	13,858	14,029	15,597	16,021	14,848	14,468
North West[2]								
Killed	538	541	522	498	512	487	468	437
Killed or seriously injured	6,219	5,579	5,391	5,172	5,334	5,470	4,972	4,811
All Casualties	33,478	34,743	35,183	36,375	39,203	40,729	39,014	40,445

1. Including Cumbria − see above text.
2. Excluding Cumbria − see above text.

1.2 Casualties

Table 1 gives the regional distribution of casualties and is presented as a time series for the period 1986 to 1992. The average for the years 1981-1985 is also given. There has been little significant change in casualty distribution over this period. In each of the seven years shown, London had the highest number of casualties. In the years 1986 to 1989 the next highest number of casualties was in the South East region but since 1990 the next highest number was in the North West region. The lowest number of casualties was in the Northern region, which, under the old regional definition, consistently had about half those in the East

Midland region, the next lowest in England. Under the revised regional definition, this proportion has fallen to about one third.

The table also shows that in 1992, as in previous years, London had the highest casualty rate per 100,000 population, followed by the North West and Eastern regions. The lowest rates were found in the Northern and South West regions. London, however, had the lowest fatality rate of all the regions - probably because accidents in urban areas tend to be less severe because they occur at lower speeds. The highest fatality rate was in the East Midlands region with the next highest in the Eastern and Yorkshire & Humberside regions.

Chart 1a depicts the number of casualties killed and the number seriously injured in each region in 1992. The chart shows that the South East and Eastern regions had the highest number of those killed and London the highest number of those seriously injured.

Chart 1b depicts the number of casualties killed and seriously injured (KSI) and slightly injured in each region in 1992 and shows that London had the highest number of casualties in both severity groups and the Northern region and Wales the lowest number.

Chart 2 depicts the number of child (aged 0-15) casualties per 100,000 child population in each region in 1992 and shows that Scotland had the highest rate of children killed and seriously injured and the South West region the lowest rate. The North West region had the highest overall rate of child casualties. **Chart 3** shows the number of adult casualties per 100,000 population in each region in 1992 and shows that Scotland and the Eastern region had the highest rate of adults killed and seriously injured and the North West region the lowest rate. The North West and London regions had the highest overall rate of adult casualties.

Charts 4 and **5** depict the percentage change in overall casualties and those killed and seriously injured for each region between 1992 and 1991 (the charts take account of the change in regional definition as noted in the introduction). **Chart 4** shows that overall casualties have fallen in six of the English regions and in Scotland and Wales. Scotland had the largest fall, at almost 5 per cent, and in England the Northern region had the largest fall, at 2½ per cent. Casualties rose in three English regions, with the North West having the largest rise, at almost 4 per cent. **Chart 5** shows that casualties killed and seriously injured fell in every English region and in Scotland and Wales. The South West region had the largest fall, at almost 9 per cent.

1.3 Local authority casualty comparisons

Tables 2-5 give information on the number of casualties, rate per 100,000 population, and percentage distribution, by age and road user type for each English county.

Table 2 gives the number of casualties by age and road user type for 1992 and **Table 3** gives the same information as an average for the years 1981-1985.

Table 4 gives casualty rates, per 100,000 population, by age and by type of road user for each English county. In England in 1992, 389 children were killed or injured in road accidents per 100,000 children and the county casualty rates varied from 256 in Avon to 568 in Merseyside. The casualty rate for those aged 60 and over varied from 153 in Avon to 356 in Surrey. The overall casualty rate for all ages was lowest in Avon and highest in Merseyside. The pedestrian casualty rate was highest in most urbanised counties, in particular

London and Greater Manchester, and lowest in rural counties such as Suffolk and Somerset. The pedal cyclist casualty rate was highest in Cambridgeshire and lowest in Durham and Northumberland. The car occupant casualty rate varied from 193 in Avon to 474 in Surrey.

Table 5 gives the distribution of casualties, by age and by type of road user, for each county. In England in 1992, 14 per cent of road accident casualties were children and 11 per cent were aged 60 and over. The proportion of casualties who were children varied from 10 per cent in Oxfordshire to 21 per cent in Cleveland. The Isle of Wight had the highest proportion of casualties aged 60 or over; 17 per cent compared with 11 per cent in the whole of England.

Table 6 gives the number of casualties killed and seriously injured and total casualties in each English county for 1992 and compares them with the average for the years 1981-1985. The percentage change is also given. In England as a whole, the number killed and seriously has fallen by 33 per cent and overall casualties by 3 per cent. The number of casualties killed and seriously injured has fallen in every county, with the largest fall, at 63 per cent, in Berkshire.

1.4 Casualties by road type

Charts 6a and **6b** depict the number of casualties killed and seriously injured and slightly injured in each region on built-up and non built-up roads respectively. On built-up roads, the highest number of casualties for both severity groups was in London, with Wales having the lowest number for both severity groups. On non built-up roads, the highest number of casualties killed and seriously injured was in the Eastern region and the highest number of slight casualties was in the South East region. The lowest number of casualties for both severity groups was in London.

Table 7 gives the total number of casualties in each region disaggregated by severity and by road type. In all regions, over 50 per cent of casualties were in accidents on built-up roads, and no more than 5 per cent in motorway accidents. The proportion of casualties who were killed and seriously injured was highest on non-built up roads.

Charts 7 and **8** show, for built-up and non built-up roads respectively, overall casualty numbers on trunk, principal and 'other' roads in each region in 1992. On built-up roads, the highest number of casualties on trunk and principal roads was in London and the highest number of casualties on 'other' roads was in the North West region. On non built-up roads, the highest number of casualties on trunk roads and 'other' roads was in the Eastern region and the highest number of casualties on principal roads in the South East region.

Table 8 gives the casualty rates by severity for motorways and A roads for each region. The casualty rate is derived by dividing the number of casualties on a particular road type by the traffic carried on those roads. The rates are given as an average for the period 1990 to 1992. The data show that the highest 'all severities' rate on motorways was in London, with the lowest in the South West region. London also had the highest 'all severities' rate for all A roads, and the South West the lowest rate. For England as a whole, the highest 'all severities' rate was on built-up trunk and principal roads, and the lowest on motorways.

1.5 Accidents

Table 9 gives accident rates by severity for motorways and A roads for each region. The accident rate is derived by dividing the number of accidents on particular road types by the traffic carried on that type of road. The rates are given as an average for the period 1990 to 1992. The data show that over the three year period, in England as a whole, built-up principal A roads had the highest overall accident rate at 103 accidents per 100 million vehicle kilometres and motorways the lowest rate at 11 accidents per 100 million vehicle kilometres. For fatal accidents, the respective rates for these two road types were 1.3 accidents and 0.3 accidents. The table also shows that accident rates were higher on principal A roads than on trunk A roads.

Chart 9 depicts the number of accidents on motorways and trunk and principal A roads in each region in 1992. The chart shows that the South East region had the highest number of accidents on motorways, and London the highest number of accidents on trunk and principal A roads.

1.6 Seasonal pattern of accidents

The seasonal pattern of injury accidents is given in **Table 10**. The base has been calculated as the average number of accidents per day in each region. The peak months for accidents can vary from year to year for various reasons, for example, differing weather conditions. The general pattern is low accident numbers in the early part of the year, gradually building up to a peak in May, June and July, followed by a small dip and then a higher peak in October and November. This trend continued in 1992, when the peak month for all accidents was November in every English region. February had the lowest number of accidents in every region. When accident figures are related to the number of days in each month, the lowest daily rate of all accidents was in February or March in all but one English region and the highest daily rate in November in every English region. The pattern for fatal and serious accidents generally follows that for all accidents, with the peak month for these accidents, in number and by day, usually varying between November and December in most regions.

1.7 Accidents by road type

Tables 11-13 show the number of junction and non-junction injury accidents occurring on motorways and trunk and principal A roads. On motorways in England, 16 per cent of accidents occurred at junctions and roundabouts. On trunk A roads, 59 per cent of accidents occurred at junctions and roundabouts as did 69 per cent of accidents on principal A roads.

Junction accidents, including those on roundabouts, accounted for about 50 per cent of all trunk A road accidents in each region except the West Midlands region where the proportion was higher at 60 per cent, and the North West and London regions, where the proportion rose to 70 and 72 per cent respectively. This pattern was repeated on principal A roads, where just over 60 per cent of accidents occurred at junctions in all regions except again in the West Midlands and North West regions where the proportion rose to 67 and 74 per cent respectively, and again in London, where the proportion was 78 per cent.

Table 14 gives the total number of injury accidents disaggregated by severity on different types of road in each region and county for 1991 and 1992. The average for the years 1981 to 1985 is also given. The road classifications used are motorways, trunk and principal A roads and all roads.

Table 15 shows injury accidents and casualties by severity, and the vehicles involved, for individual English motorways, including A(M) roads. Eighty two per cent of the vehicles involved were cars or vans while 14 per cent were heavy lorries, broadly in line with their share of motorway traffic. Motorways with the highest numbers of accidents per kilometre in 1992 were the M25 (4 accidents), the M63 (3.5), and the M4 (3.1 accidents).

Table 16 gives the percentage of accidents on the various types of road within each region. This table should be considered in conjunction with Table 19 which shows the distribution of motor traffic within each region.

1.8 Background data

Table 17 gives regional background information on road lengths, home population, area, and licensed vehicle numbers. **Table 18** gives the 1990-1992 average distribution between regions of motor traffic on major roads, and **Table 19** shows the distribution of motor traffic within each region. The English motorway lengths shown in Tables 15 and 17 have been supplied by DOT Highways Computing Division from data extracted from the Network Information System (NIS). Other road lengths in Table 17 are taken from the Transport Statistics Report 'Road Lengths in Great Britain 1992'.

List of charts and tables   Page

Charts

Tables

CHARTS

Chart 1a: Fatal and serious casualties: by region: 1992

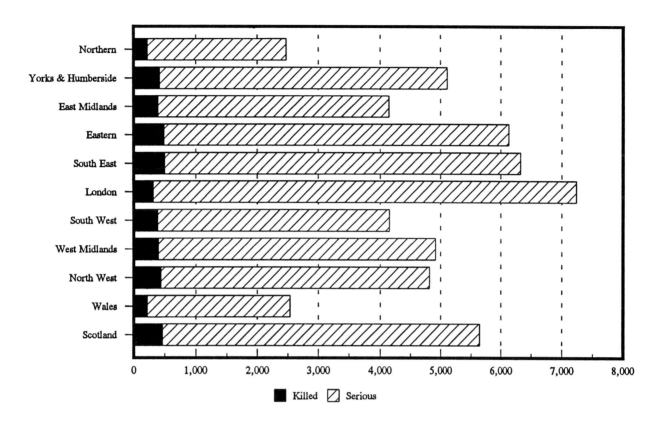

Killed ■ Serious ▨

Chart 1b: KSI and slight casualties: by region: 1992

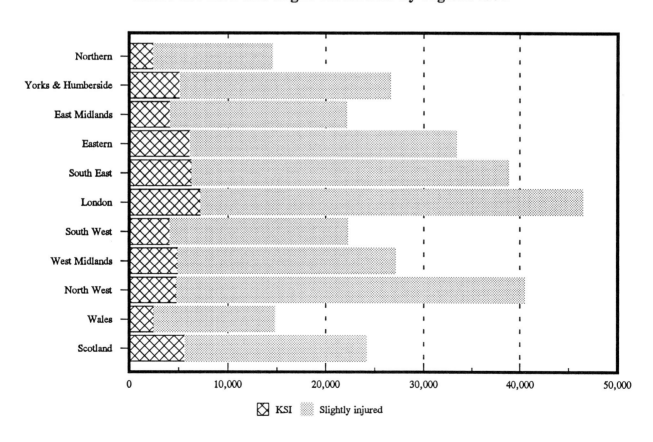

⊠ KSI ░ Slightly injured

Chart 2: Child casualties per 100,000 population: by severity and region: 1992

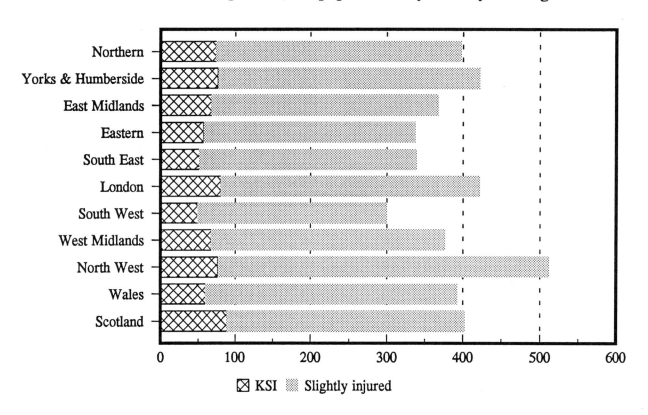

Chart 3: Adult casualties per 100,000 population: by severity and region: 1992

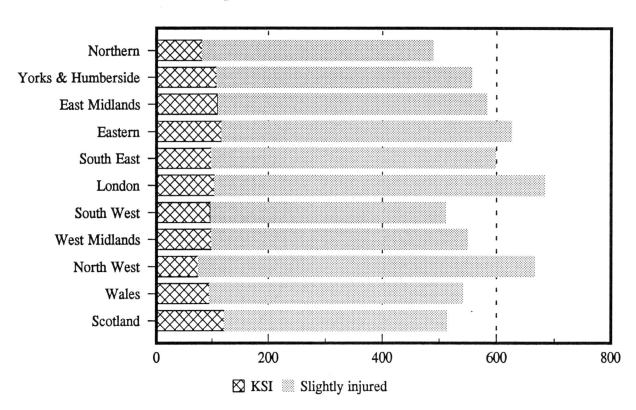

Chart 4: Percentage change in total casualties: by region: 1991-1992

Percentage change

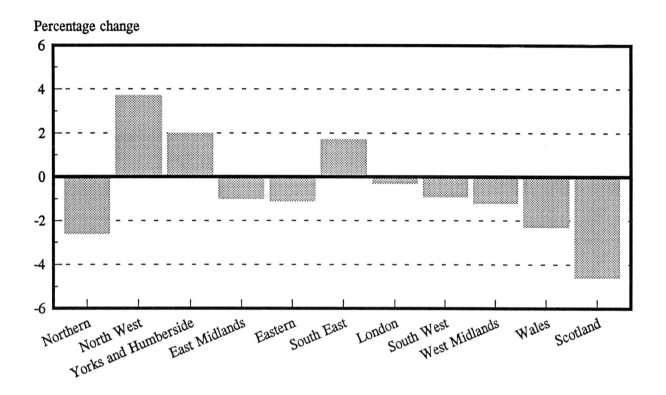

Chart 5: Percentage change in KSI casualties: by region: 1991-1992

Percentage change

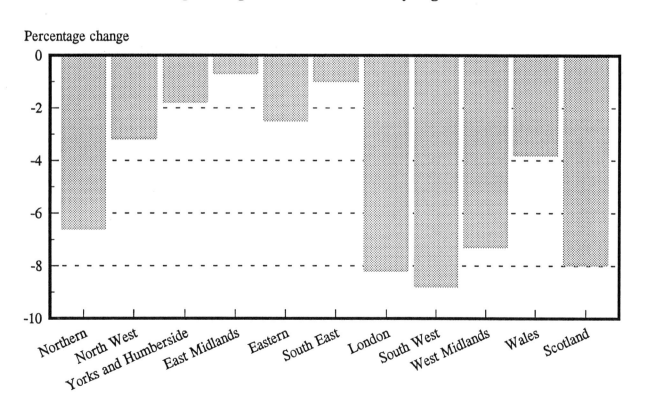

Chart 6a: Casualties on built-up roads: by severity and region: 1992

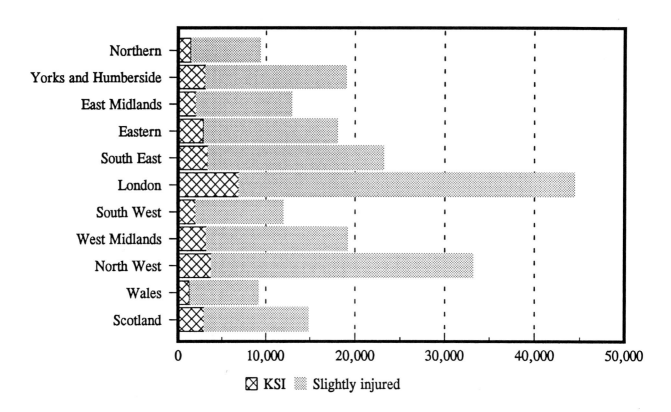

KSI   Slightly injured

Chart 6b: Casualties on non built-up roads: by severity and region: 1992

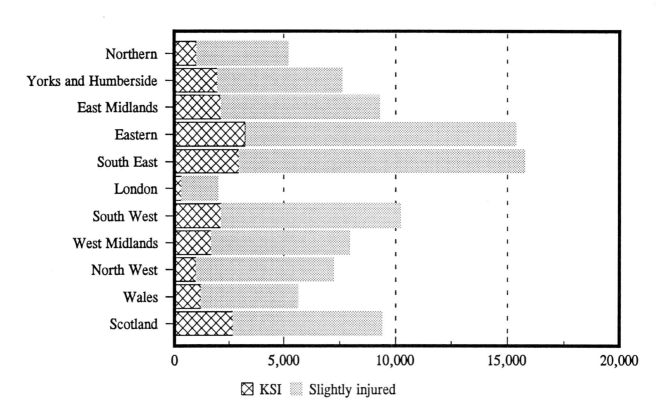

KSI   Slightly injured

Chart 7: Casualties by road class and region: built-up roads: 1992

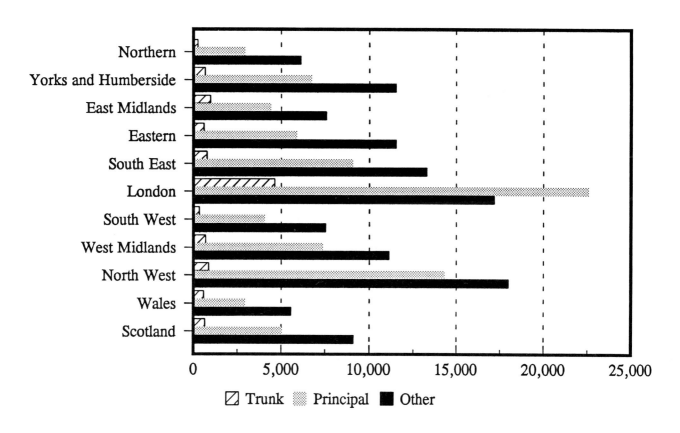

Trunk · Principal ■ Other

Chart 8: Casualties by road class and region: non built-up roads: 1992

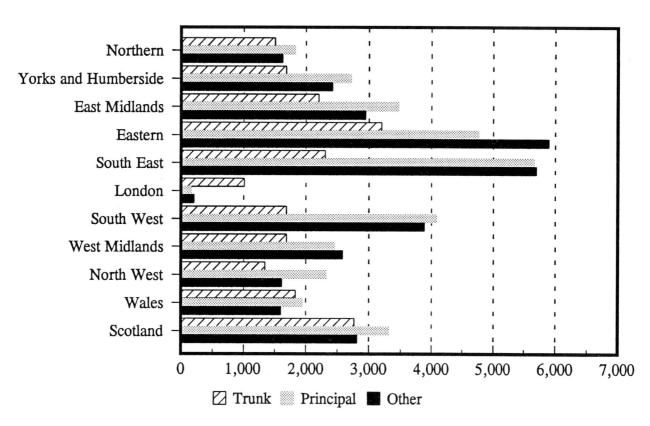

Trunk · Principal ■ Other

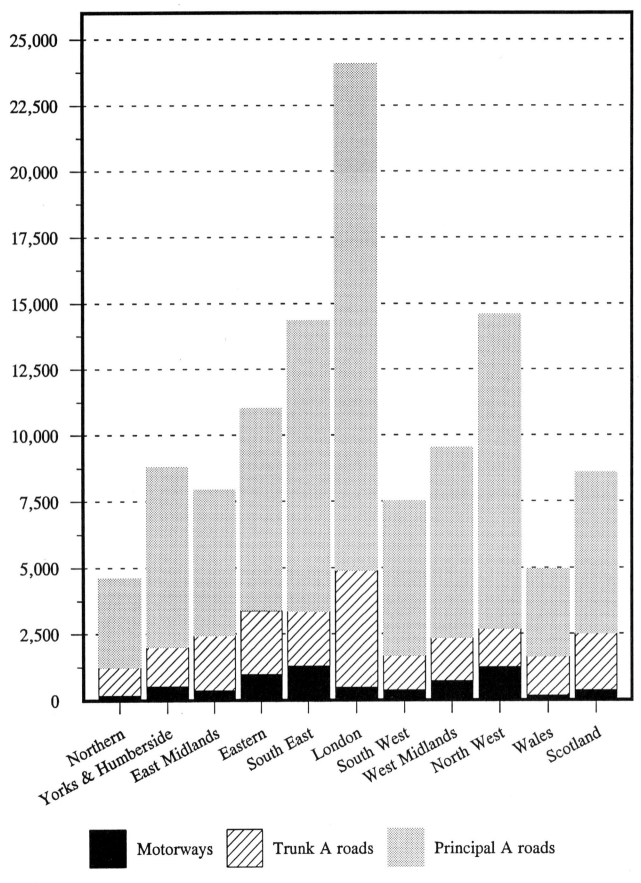

Chart 9: Accidents by road class and region: 1992

Motorways   Trunk A roads   Principal A roads

TABLES

1 Casualties: by region and severity: 1981-85 average, 1986-1992: rate per 100,000 population, 1992

Number/rate

	1981-85 Average	1986	1987	1988	1989	1990	1991	1992	1992 Rate Per 100,000 Population[1]
Northern[2]									
Killed	282	261	294	280	270	334	287	225	7.3
Killed or seriously injured	3,566	3,158	2,916	2,947	2,962	3,050	2,651	2,475	80.1
All Casualties	13,913	13,783	13,858	14,029	15,597	16,021	14,848	14,468	468.0
Yorkshire and Humberside									
Killed	501	499	440	437	480	428	413	414	8.3
Killed or seriously injured	6,830	6,559	5,817	6,131	6,127	5,978	5,202	5,110	102.6
All Casualties	25,915	25,922	25,328	26,884	28,560	28,455	26,086	26,599	533.8
East Midlands									
Killed	492	458	448	413	514	513	410	393	9.7
Killed or seriously injured	6,389	5,516	5,254	5,031	5,342	5,045	4,173	4,145	102.7
All Casualties	23,079	22,819	22,494	23,308	25,129	24,852	22,397	22,175	549.5
Eastern									
Killed	601	606	614	587	617	608	546	488	8.4
Killed or seriously injured	9,312	8,734	8,318	8,230	7,967	7,653	6,287	6,132	105.9
All Casualties	33,789	36,527	35,886	37,896	39,424	37,908	33,768	33,388	576.8
South East									
Killed	735	698	676	718	715	699	516	496	7.0
Killed or seriously injured	11,038	10,134	9,446	9,321	8,766	8,155	6,388	6,325	89.8
All Casualties	41,999	41,920	40,326	41,184	43,050	42,387	38,211	38,876	552.2
London[3]									
Killed	539	520	456	446	460	408	368	316	4.6
Killed or seriously injured	8,230 (9,175)	8,798	9,517	9,478	9,344	8,910	7,878	7,233	105.0
All Casualties	54,156	51,610	49,454	50,114	52,779	51,871	46,578	46,417	673.7
South West									
Killed	484	459	457	462	521	468	460	385	8.2
Killed or seriously injured	8,047	7,305	6,250	6,134	5,781	5,424	4,555	4,153	88.0
All Casualties	26,352	26,178	24,507	25,444	25,246	25,034	22,515	22,302	472.7
West Midlands									
Killed	526	506	442	442	498	478	386	395	7.5
Killed or seriously injured	7,857	6,853	5,860	5,774	6,190	6,136	5,298	4,913	93.3
All Casualties	27,699	27,409	25,425	26,760	28,964	30,219	27,425	27,089	514.5
North West[2]									
Killed	538	541	522	498	512	487	468	437	6.8
Killed or seriously injured	6,219	5,579	5,391	5,172	5,334	5,470	4,972	4,811	75.2
All Casualties	33,478	34,743	35,183	36,375	39,203	40,729	39,014	40,445	632.3
England									
Killed	4,698	4,546	4,349	4,283	4,587	4,423	3,854	3,549	7.4
Killed or seriously injured	67,388	62,636	58,769	58,218	57,813	55,821	47,404	45,297	94.0
All Casualties	280,382	280,895	272,461	281,994	297,952	297,476	270,842	271,759	563.7
Wales									
Killed	259	235	220	226	233	249	227	220	7.6
Killed or seriously injured	3,855	3,478	3,388	3,127	3,191	3,037	2,638	2,537	87.7
All Casualties	14,395	14,446	14,266	15,164	16,165	16,432	15,074	14,732	509.5
Scotland									
Killed	641	601	556	543	553	545	487	460	9.3
Killed or seriously injured	8,887	8,022	7,261	7,198	7,527	6,800	6,131	5,640	114.6
All Casualties	27,134	26,110	24,746	25,147	27,475	27,233	25,353	24,182	491.4
Great Britain									
Killed	5,598	5,382	5,125	5,052	5,373	5,217	4,568	4,229	7.5
Killed or seriously injured	80,130	74,134	69,418	68,543	68,531	65,658	56,173	53,474	95.5
All Casualties	321,912	321,451	311,473	322,305	341,592	341,141	311,269	310,673	554.6
Northern Ireland									
Killed	196	236	214	178	181	185	185	150	9.4
Killed or seriously injured	2,362	2,061	2,099	2,147	2,195	2,178	1,833	1,991	124.9
All Casualties	8,204	9,442	9,936	10,967	11,611	11,761	10,314	11,264	706.5
United Kingdom									
Killed	5,793	5,618	5,339	5,230	5,554	5,402	4,753	4,379	7.6
Killed or seriously injured	82,492	76,195	71,517	70,690	70,726	67,836	58,006	55,465	96.3
All Casualties	330,115	330,893	321,409	333,272	353,203	352,902	321,583	321,937	558.8

1 Final 1991 population estimates were used for England, Wales and Scotland. Provisional 1991 estimates were used for Northern Ireland.
2 From 1st April 1991 responsibilty for Cumbria transferred from the North West Regional Office to the Northern Regional Office. The change to the road accident database was deferred until 1992. Data prior to 1992 for both Northern and North West regions have been revised to take account of the change in boundaries (see introduction on page 3).
3. In September 1984 the Metropolitan Police implemented revised standards in the assessment of serious casualties. The figure in brackets are an estimate of casualty totals under standards prevailing since 1984. See notes.

2 Number of casualties: by county, by type of road user: 1992

	Children (0-15)	Adults (16-59)	Older adults (60+)	All[1] casualties	Pedest- rians	Pedal cyclists	Motor cyclists	Car occupants	Other[2] road users
Avon	473	2,604	315	3,409	585	331	438	1,860	195
Bedfordshire	405	2,285	267	2,958	391	235	253	1,859	220
Berkshire	467	2,787	333	3,735	461	375	334	2,393	172
Buckinghamshire	479	2,930	305	3,851	369	241	364	2,626	251
Cambridgeshire	560	3,628	436	4,656	359	729	433	2,827	308
Cheshire	776	4,189	551	5,516	628	469	425	3,640	354
Cleveland	550	1,839	236	2,625	605	221	119	1,490	190
Cornwall	295	1,848	300	2,443	254	128	265	1,640	156
Cumbria	350	1,901	282	2,533	351	160	242	1,627	153
Derbyshire	622	3,741	455	5,004	670	317	495	3,316	206
Devon	601	3,557	671	4,829	698	332	632	2,945	222
Dorset	396	2,568	473	3,437	370	246	336	2,309	176
Durham	474	2,187	248	2,917	539	132	149	1,834	263
East Sussex	454	2,647	538	3,639	584	277	325	2,202	251
Essex	926	6,307	818	8,469	944	674	715	5,660	476
Gloucestershire	334	2,106	327	2,767	324	261	328	1,735	119
Greater London	5,656	33,277	4,462	46,417	9,854	4,274	5,594	22,494	4,201
Greater Manchester	3,013	12,000	1,486	16,500	3,665	1,334	824	9,626	1,051
Hampshire	1,032	6,643	925	8,600	967	966	999	5,193	475
Hereford & Worcester	444	2,588	358	3,390	404	312	349	2,159	166
Hertfordshire	678	4,214	503	5,452	581	434	430	3,672	335
Humberside	814	3,413	493	5,030	855	706	623	2,468	378
Isle of Wight	80	407	96	583	111	48	71	325	28
Kent	1,109	6,184	839	8,220	1,151	634	933	5,034	468
Lancashire	1,373	6,005	864	8,288	1,568	664	629	4,870	557
Leicestershire	650	3,563	427	4,640	641	437	433	2,849	280
Lincolnshire	466	2,739	380	3,585	318	297	330	2,384	256
Merseyside	1,735	7,353	1,053	10,141	1,877	626	399	6,549	690
Norfolk	548	3,644	599	4,871	453	440	531	3,177	270
Northamptonshire	405	2,372	289	3,071	405	198	280	2,015	173
Northumberland	201	1,200	174	1,575	180	68	89	1,077	161
North Yorkshire	539	3,513	536	4,600	432	376	460	3,006	326
Nottinghamshire	857	4,172	515	5,875	908	537	568	3,419	443
Oxfordshire	319	2,497	319	3,298	283	346	325	2,104	240
Shropshire	276	1,696	222	2,194	201	157	192	1,554	90
Somerset	247	1,638	277	2,313	227	204	218	1,512	152
South Yorkshire	1,000	4,205	653	5,858	1,228	380	369	3,336	545
Staffordshire	792	5,067	604	6,463	806	405	515	4,374	363
Suffolk	397	2,358	374	3,131	281	338	387	1,943	182
Surrey	761	5,528	781	7,133	636	627	639	4,902	329
Tyne & Wear	920	3,357	541	4,818	1,251	352	186	2,623	406
Warwickshire	369	2,366	315	3,176	303	265	265	2,106	237
West Midlands	2,243	8,358	1,265	11,866	2,945	873	765	6,585	698
West Sussex	461	2,731	476	3,668	427	353	330	2,330	228
West Yorkshire	1,920	7,972	1,219	11,111	2,402	673	727	6,391	918
Wiltshire	345	2,424	334	3,104	303	234	312	2,016	239
England	37,812	200,608	27,934	271,759	43,795	22,686	24,625	162,056	18,597
Wales	2,323	10,757	1,651	14,732	2,435	775	1,012	9,605	905
Scotland	4,051	17,265	2,825	24,182	5,357	1,294	1,236	13,984	2,311
Great Britain	44,186	228,630	32,410	310,673	51,587	24,755	26,873	185,645	21,813
Northern Ireland	1,667	8,661	936	11,264	1,347	386	348	8,209	974
United Kingdom	45,853	237,291	33,346	321,937	52,934	25,141	27,221	193,854	22,787

Number of casualties

1 Includes age not reported.
2 Includes road user type not known.

24

3 Number of casualties: by county, by type of road user: 1981-1985 average[1]

	Children (0-15)	Adults (16-59)	Older adults (60+)	All[2] casualties	Pedest-rians	Pedal cyclists	Motor cyclists	Car occupants	Other[3] road users
Avon	616	3,520	447	4,584	777	402	1,399	1,768	238
Bedfordshire	502	2,480	252	3,235	495	299	628	1,552	262
Berkshire	573	3,232	333	4,243	567	449	904	2,167	157
Buckinghamshire	464	2,713	283	3,504	409	287	700	1,940	168
Cambridgeshire	489	3,095	397	3,981	345	646	923	1,834	233
Cheshire	803	3,789	490	5,095	711	593	1,126	2,324	341
Cleveland	587	1,853	231	2,671	682	274	515	1,016	185
Cornwall	359	2,079	253	2,691	339	151	756	1,301	144
Cumbria	441	2,068	297	2,806	444	216	606	1,383	157
Derbyshire	715	3,505	439	4,933	808	405	1,207	2,098	415
Devon	769	4,333	624	5,726	845	400	1,654	2,526	302
Dorset	461	2,745	471	3,677	487	396	959	1,647	188
Durham	450	1,806	221	2,476	510	140	412	1,216	198
East Sussex	535	2,722	655	3,911	725	287	830	1,842	227
Essex	1,344	7,165	947	9,474	1,212	803	1,845	5,003	611
Gloucestershire	419	2,549	308	3,276	378	348	926	1,465	160
Greater London	7,106	37,831	5,855	54,156	13,081	4,739	9,957	21,778	4,601
Greater Manchester	2,946	9,320	1,431	13,699	3,931	1,376	2,284	5,186	922
Hampshire	1,276	7,151	881	9,308	1,159	1,182	2,530	3,981	456
Hereford & Worcester	491	2,895	384	3,770	461	370	847	1,909	183
Hertfordshire	784	4,401	485	5,729	738	511	1,173	3,003	304
Humberside	842	3,601	491	4,934	821	727	1,377	1,620	388
Isle of Wight	107	481	74	662	107	61	206	260	28
Kent	1,251	6,769	848	8,867	1,246	744	2,291	4,139	447
Lancashire	1,399	5,155	906	7,460	1,683	666	1,458	3,188	466
Leicestershire	752	3,657	415	4,825	827	507	1,117	2,124	249
Lincolnshire	501	2,866	382	3,749	365	381	852	1,929	221
Merseyside	1,632	4,718	875	7,225	2,066	583	1,009	2,926	642
Norfolk	551	3,195	495	4,241	483	456	1,063	1,999	240
Northamptonshire	499	2,818	334	3,652	449	240	779	1,913	271
Northumberland	215	1,142	159	1,516	192	95	270	828	131
North Yorkshire	568	3,349	496	4,413	531	420	1,030	2,150	283
Nottinghamshire	987	4,364	570	5,920	1,111	609	1,362	2,381	458
Oxfordshire	389	2,677	297	3,424	362	382	798	1,663	219
Shropshire	297	1,767	211	2,275	252	185	473	1,237	129
Somerset	299	1,875	276	2,450	267	222	640	1,204	117
South Yorkshire	1,108	4,121	685	5,914	1,475	354	1,069	2,308	708
Staffordshire	1,038	4,972	518	6,528	983	558	1,388	3,167	432
Suffolk	479	2,762	385	3,627	397	389	961	1,696	183
Surrey	921	5,844	779	7,640	808	838	1,764	3,918	312
Tyne & Wear	1,028	2,906	509	4,443	1,491	334	650	1,568	400
Warwickshire	400	2,179	261	2,839	339	295	606	1,446	154
West Midlands	2,714	8,345	1,227	12,286	3,596	1,064	1,993	4,812	820
West Sussex	498	2,919	527	3,943	440	464	907	1,953	180
West Yorkshire	2,039	7,531	1,084	10,654	2,728	722	2,048	4,386	770
Wiltshire	491	3,080	377	3,948	392	358	887	2,056	256
England	43,133	204,343	28,867	280,382	52,515	25,927	59,179	123,806	18,956
Wales	2,320	10,500	1,576	14,395	2,666	857	2,566	7,211	1,094
Scotland	4,881	19,157	3,097	27,134	6,560	1,607	3,446	12,924	2,598
Great Britain	50,334	234,000	33,540	321,912	61,741	28,391	65,191	143,941	22,647
Northern Ireland[4]	1,516	5,954	731	8,204	1,648	399	765	5,398	
United Kingdom[4]	51,850	239,954	34,271	330,115	63,389	28,791	65,956	171,986	

1 Figures have been rounded so there may be an apparent slight discrepancy between the sum of the constituent items and the total as shown
2 Includes age not reported.
3 Includes road user type not known.
4 It is not possible to give separate casualty figures for car occupants and other road users for Northern Ireland for these years.

4 Total casualty rates[1] : by county, by type of road user: 1992

	Children (0-15)	Adults (16-59)	Older adults (60+)	All[2] casualties	Pedest-rians	Pedal cyclists	Motor cyclists	Car occupants	Other[3] road users
Avon	256	454	153	353	61	34	45	193	20
Bedfordshire	341	705	298	556	73	44	48	349	41
Berkshire	294	594	267	496	61	50	44	318	23
Buckinghamshire	340	748	286	603	58	38	57	411	39
Cambridgeshire	408	893	349	696	54	109	65	423	46
Cheshire	387	731	287	571	65	49	44	377	37
Cleveland	435	563	221	469	108	39	21	266	34
Cornwall	324	704	249	515	54	27	56	346	33
Cumbria	371	672	252	518	72	33	49	333	31
Derbyshire	333	674	226	531	71	34	52	352	22
Devon	313	612	253	465	67	32	61	284	21
Dorset	341	719	253	520	56	37	51	350	27
Durham	390	615	193	482	89	22	25	303	43
East Sussex	363	682	266	509	82	39	45	308	35
Essex	297	694	251	547	61	44	46	366	31
Gloucestershire	316	671	273	513	60	48	61	322	22
Greater London	422	778	350	674	143	62	81	326	61
Greater Manchester	550	795	290	642	143	52	32	374	41
Hampshire	326	700	292	544	61	61	63	328	30
Hereford & Worcester	319	647	245	495	59	46	51	315	24
Hertfordshire	337	708	262	551	59	44	43	371	34
Humberside	447	670	266	573	97	80	71	281	43
Isle of Wight	348	611	261	461	88	38	56	257	22
Kent	354	692	255	535	75	41	61	328	30
Lancashire	470	744	277	588	111	47	45	345	40
Leicestershire	347	668	246	519	72	49	48	319	31
Lincolnshire	410	814	270	607	54	50	56	403	43
Merseyside	568	880	341	700	129	43	28	452	48
Norfolk	388	845	321	641	60	58	70	418	36
Northamptonshire	318	681	260	524	69	34	48	343	29
Northumberland	328	678	254	514	59	22	29	351	52
North Yorkshire	399	839	325	640	60	52	64	418	45
Nottinghamshire	421	687	246	576	89	53	56	335	43
Oxfordshire	273	696	303	568	49	60	56	362	41
Shropshire	324	702	262	533	49	38	47	378	22
Somerset	267	627	242	494	48	44	47	323	32
South Yorkshire	391	545	238	450	94	29	28	256	42
Staffordshire	370	803	295	616	77	39	49	417	35
Suffolk	296	632	255	479	43	52	59	297	28
Surrey	386	895	356	690	62	61	62	474	32
Tyne & Wear	407	508	222	426	111	31	16	232	36
Warwickshire	380	813	312	649	62	54	54	431	48
West Midlands	400	545	236	451	112	33	29	250	27
West Sussex	348	697	253	515	60	50	46	327	32
West Yorkshire	437	648	294	533	115	32	35	307	44
Wiltshire	295	713	290	543	53	41	55	353	42
England	389	705	279	564	91	47	51	336	39
Wales	80	652	254	510	84	27	35	332	31
Scotland	402	590	286	491	109	26	25	284	47
Great Britain	391	692	278	555	92	44	48	331	39
Northern Ireland	404	952	345	706	84	24	22	515	61
United Kingdom	391	699	279	559	92	44	47	336	40

1 Final 1991 population estimates were used for England, Wales and Scotland. Provisional 1991 estimates were used for Northern Ireland.
2 Includes age not reported.
3 Includes road user type not known.

5 Casualty indicators: by county, by type of road user: 1992

Percentage of all casualties

	Children[1] (0-15)	Adults[1] (16-59)	Older adults[1] (60+)	Pedest- rians	Pedal cyclists	Motor cyclists	Car occupants	Other[2] road users
Avon	13.9	76.8	9.3	17.2	9.7	12.8	54.6	5.7
Bedfordshire	13.7	77.3	9.0	13.2	7.9	8.6	62.8	7.4
Berkshire	13.0	77.7	9.3	12.3	10.0	8.9	64.1	4.6
Buckinghamshire	12.9	78.9	8.2	9.6	6.3	9.5	68.2	6.5
Cambridgeshire	12.1	78.5	9.4	7.7	15.7	9.3	60.7	6.6
Cheshire	14.1	75.9	10.0	11.4	8.5	7.7	66.0	6.4
Cleveland	21.0	70.1	9.0	23.0	8.4	4.5	56.8	7.2
Cornwall	12.1	75.6	12.3	10.4	5.2	10.8	67.1	6.4
Cumbria	13.8	75.0	11.1	13.9	6.3	9.6	64.2	6.0
Derbyshire	12.9	77.6	9.4	13.4	6.3	9.9	66.3	4.1
Devon	12.4	73.7	13.9	14.5	6.9	13.1	61.0	4.6
Dorset	11.5	74.7	13.8	10.8	7.2	9.8	67.2	5.1
Durham	16.3	75.2	8.5	18.5	4.5	5.1	62.9	9.0
East Sussex	12.5	72.7	14.8	16.0	7.6	8.9	60.5	6.9
Essex	11.5	78.3	10.2	11.1	8.0	8.4	66.8	5.6
Gloucestershire	12.1	76.1	11.8	11.7	9.4	11.9	62.7	4.3
Greater London	13.0	76.7	10.3	21.2	9.2	12.1	48.5	9.1
Greater Manchester	18.3	72.7	9.0	22.2	8.1	5.0	58.3	6.4
Hampshire	12.0	77.2	10.8	11.2	11.2	11.6	60.4	5.5
Hereford & Worcester	13.1	76.3	10.6	11.9	9.2	10.3	63.7	4.9
Hertfordshire	12.6	78.1	9.3	10.7	8.0	7.9	67.4	6.1
Humberside	17.2	72.3	10.4	17.0	14.0	12.4	49.1	7.5
Isle of Wight	13.7	69.8	16.5	19.0	8.2	12.2	55.7	4.8
Kent	13.6	76.0	10.3	14.0	7.7	11.4	61.2	5.7
Lancashire	16.7	72.9	10.5	18.9	8.0	7.6	58.8	6.7
Leicestershire	14.0	76.8	9.2	13.8	9.4	9.3	61.4	6.0
Lincolnshire	13.0	76.4	10.6	8.9	8.3	9.2	66.5	7.1
Merseyside	17.1	72.5	10.4	18.5	6.2	3.9	64.6	6.8
Norfolk	11.4	76.1	12.5	9.3	9.0	10.9	65.2	5.5
Northamptonshire	13.2	77.4	9.4	13.2	6.4	9.1	65.6	5.6
Northumberland	12.8	76.2	11.0	11.4	4.3	5.7	68.4	10.2
North Yorkshire	11.7	76.6	11.7	9.4	8.2	10.0	65.3	7.1
Nottinghamshire	15.5	75.3	9.3	15.5	9.1	9.7	58.2	7.5
Oxfordshire	10.2	79.6	10.2	8.6	10.5	9.9	63.8	7.3
Shropshire	12.6	77.3	10.1	9.2	7.2	8.8	70.8	4.1
Somerset	11.4	75.8	12.8	9.8	8.8	9.4	65.4	6.6
South Yorkshire	17.1	71.8	11.1	21.0	6.5	6.3	56.9	9.3
Staffordshire	12.3	78.4	9.3	12.5	6.3	8.0	67.7	5.6
Suffolk	12.7	75.4	12.0	9.0	10.8	12.4	62.1	5.8
Surrey	10.8	78.2	11.0	8.9	8.8	9.0	68.7	4.6
Tyne & Wear	19.1	69.7	11.2	26.0	7.3	3.9	54.4	8.4
Warwickshire	12.1	77.6	10.3	9.5	8.3	8.3	66.3	7.5
West Midlands	18.9	70.4	10.7	24.8	7.4	6.4	55.5	5.9
West Sussex	12.6	74.5	13.0	11.6	9.6	9.0	63.5	6.2
West Yorkshire	17.3	71.7	11.0	21.6	6.1	6.5	57.5	8.3
Wiltshire	11.1	78.1	10.8	9.8	7.5	10.1	64.9	7.7
England	14.2	75.3	10.5	16.1	8.3	9.1	59.6	6.8
Wales	15.8	73.0	11.2	16.5	5.3	6.9	65.2	6.1
Scotland	16.8	71.5	11.7	22.2	5.4	5.1	57.8	9.6
Great Britain	14.5	74.9	10.6	16.6	8.0	8.6	59.8	7.0
Northern Ireland	14.8	76.9	8.3	12.0	3.4	3.1	72.9	8.6
United Kingdom	14.2	73.7	10.4	16.4	7.8	8.5	60.2	7.1

Percentage of all casualties who are:

1 Percentage of casualties of known age.
2 Includes road user type not known.

6 Casualty changes: by county and severity: 1981-1985 average, 1992

	Killed and seriously injured			All casualties		
	Average 1981-1985	1992	percentage change	Average 1981-1985	1992	percentage change
Avon	1,356	582	*-57.1*	4,584	3,409	*-25.6*
Bedfordshire	714	442	*-38.1*	3,235	2,958	*-8.6*
Berkshire	1,095	406	*-62.9*	4,243	3,735	*-12.0*
Buckinghamshire	1,031	484	*-53.1*	3,504	3,851	*9.9*
Cambridgeshire	1,087	995	*-8.4*	3,981	4,656	*17.0*
Cheshire	916	643	*-29.8*	5,095	5,516	*8.3*
Cleveland	486	369	*-24.1*	2,671	2,625	*-1.7*
Cornwall	858	473	*-44.8*	2,691	2,443	*-9.2*
Cumbria	829	565	*-31.8*	2,806	2,533	*-9.7*
Derbyshire	1,222	672	*-45.0*	4,933	5,004	*1.4*
Devon	1,897	1,010	*-46.8*	5,726	4,829	*-15.7*
Dorset	940	526	*-44.1*	3,677	3,437	*-6.5*
Durham	703	425	*-39.6*	2,476	2,917	*17.8*
East Sussex	989	569	*-42.5*	3,911	3,639	*-7.0*
Essex	2,398	1,312	*-45.3*	9,474	8,469	*-10.6*
Gloucestershire	1,166	466	*-60.0*	3,276	2,767	*-15.5*
Greater London[1]	8,230 (9,175)	7,233	*-12.1*	54,156	46,417	*-14.3*
Greater Manchester	2,362	1,752	*-25.8*	13,699	16,500	*20.4*
Hampshire	2,755	1,593	*-42.2*	9,308	8,600	*-7.6*
Hereford & Worcester	1,071	610	*-43.1*	3,770	3,390	*-10.1*
Hertfordshire	1,388	1,054	*-24.0*	5,729	5,452	*-4.8*
Humberside	1,129	984	*-12.8*	4,934	5,030	*2.0*
Isle of Wight	184	130	*-29.3*	662	583	*-11.9*
Kent	2,385	1,534	*-35.7*	8,867	8,220	*-7.3*
Lancashire	1,704	1,346	*-21.0*	7,460	8,288	*11.1*
Leicestershire	1,226	714	*-41.8*	4,825	4,640	*-3.8*
Lincolnshire	1,074	819	*-23.7*	3,749	3,585	*-4.4*
Merseyside	1,237	1,070	*-13.5*	7,225	10,141	*40.4*
Norfolk	1,524	1,130	*-25.9*	4,241	4,871	*14.9*
Northamptonshire	1,328	744	*-44.0*	3,652	3,071	*-15.9*
Northumberland	400	289	*-27.7*	1,516	1,575	*3.9*
North Yorkshire	1,835	1,358	*-26.0*	4,413	4,600	*4.2*
Nottinghamshire	1,540	1,196	*-22.3*	5,920	5,875	*-0.8*
Oxfordshire	1,067	532	*-50.2*	3,424	3,298	*-3.7*
Shropshire	833	526	*-36.9*	2,275	2,194	*-3.6*
Somerset	811	470	*-42.0*	2,450	2,313	*-5.6*
South Yorkshire	1,320	845	*-36.0*	5,914	5,858	*-0.9*
Staffordshire	1,442	736	*-49.0*	6,528	6,463	*-1.0*
Suffolk	1,170	715	*-38.9*	3,627	3,131	*-13.7*
Surrey	1,641	1,013	*-38.3*	7,640	7,133	*-6.6*
Tyne & Wear	1,048	827	*-21.1*	4,443	4,818	*8.4*
Warwickshire	1,059	836	*-21.1*	2,839	3,176	*11.9*
West Midlands	3,452	2,205	*-36.1*	12,286	11,866	*-3.4*
West Sussex	922	548	*-40.6*	3,943	3,668	*-7.0*
West Yorkshire	2,547	1,923	*-24.5*	10,654	11,111	*4.3*
Wiltshire	1,019	626	*-38.6*	3,948	3,104	*-21.4*
England	67,388	45,297	*-32.8*	280,382	271,759	*-3.1*
Wales	3,855	2,537	*-34.2*	14,395	14,732	*2.3*
Scotland	8,887	5,640	*-36.5*	27,134	24,182	*-10.9*
Great Britain	80,130	53,474	*-33.3*	321,912	310,673	*-3.5*
Northern Ireland	2,362	1,991	*-15.7*	8,204	11,264	*37.3*
United Kingdom	82,492	55,465	*-32.8*	330,115	321,937	*-2.5*

1 In September 1984 the Metropolitan Police implemented revised standards in the assessment of serious casualties.
The figure in brackets is an estimate of casualty totals under standards prevailing since 1984. See notes.

7 Number of casualties: by road class, region[1] and severity: 1992

	Motorways	Built up				Non built up				All roads[2]
		Trunk	Principal	Other	Total	Trunk	Principal	Other	Total	
Northern[3]										
Killed	8	1	20	57	78	53	60	26	139	225
Killed or Seriously Injured	42	35	410	1,004	1,449	290	390	304	984	2,475
All Casualties	252	252	2,896	6,120	9,268	1,503	1,822	1,623	4,948	14,468
Yorkshire and Humberside										
Killed	18	7	87	112	206	45	91	54	190	414
Killed or Seriously Injured	146	98	1,084	1,932	3,114	476	760	612	1,848	5,110
All Casualties	863	668	6,739	11,510	18,917	1,681	2,708	2,421	6,810	26,599
East Midlands										
Killed	22	12	49	56	117	85	91	78	254	393
Killed or Seriously Injured	121	158	636	1,210	2,004	503	822	693	2,018	4,145
All Casualties	636	966	4,377	7,568	12,911	2,200	3,470	2,949	8,619	22,175
Eastern										
Killed	28	6	44	88	138	83	144	95	322	488
Killed or Seriously Injured	216	89	885	1,898	2,872	660	1,056	1,328	3,044	6,132
All Casualties	1,520	599	5,894	11,521	18,014	3,194	4,760	5,897	13,851	33,388
South East										
Killed	49	8	73	103	184	53	121	89	263	496
Killed or Seriously Injured	305	124	1,298	1,941	3,363	393	1,131	1,133	2,657	6,325
All Casualties	2,090	772	9,078	13,272	23,122	2,303	5,663	5,698	13,664	38,876
London										
Killed	4	53	137	106	296	11	1	4	16	316
Killed or Seriously Injured	83	679	3,490	2,733	6,902	178	26	44	248	7,233
All Casualties	677	4,629	22,565	17,170	44,364	1,009	158	209	1,376	46,417
South West										
Killed	19	4	55	70	129	63	104	70	237	385
Killed or Seriously Injured	109	42	688	1,245	1,975	329	894	818	2,041	4,153
All Casualties	617	335	4,022	7,545	11,902	1,685	4,072	3,884	9,641	22,302
West Midlands										
Killed	29	16	97	97	210	54	61	41	156	395
Killed or Seriously Injured	201	114	1,194	1,905	3,213	386	531	582	1,499	4,913
All Casualties	1,203	696	7,367	11,104	19,167	1,688	2,450	2,581	6,719	27,089
North West[3]										
Killed	42	8	154	132	294	32	46	23	101	437
Killed or Seriously Injured	210	85	1,582	2,123	3,790	180	402	228	810	4,811
All Casualties	1,983	861	14,299	18,015	33,175	1,340	2,322	1,611	5,273	40,445
England										
Killed	219	115	716	821	1,652	479	719	480	1,678	3,549
Killed or Seriously Injured	1,433	1,424	11,267	15,991	28,682	3,395	6,012	5,742	15,149	45,297
All Casualties	9,841	9,778	77,237	103,825	190,840	16,603	27,425	26,873	70,901	271,759
Wales										
Killed	3	11	37	59	107	52	39	19	110	220
Killed or Seriously Injured	36	105	413	785	1,303	440	437	321	1,198	2,537
All Casualties	268	582	2,945	5,565	9,092	1,831	1,942	1,599	5,372	14,732
Scotland										
Killed	16	13	62	90	165	122	98	59	279	460
Killed or Seriously Injured	107	131	1,006	1,824	2,961	872	943	757	2,572	5,640
All Casualties	513	657	5,013	9,109	14,779	2,768	3,306	2,816	8,890	24,182
Great Britain										
Killed	238	139	815	970	1,924	653	856	558	2,067	4,229
Killed or Seriously Injured	1,576	1,660	12,686	18,600	32,946	4,707	7,392	6,820	18,919	53,474
All Casualties	10,622	11,017	85,195	118,499	214,711	21,202	32,673	31,288	85,163	310,673

1 Casualty data by road class are not available for Northern Ireland.
2 Includes speed limit not reported.
3 From 1st April 1991 responsibilty for Cumbria transferred from the North West Regional Office to the Northern Regional Office.
   The change to the road accident database was deferred until 1992. Consequently data prior to 1992 for both Northern and North West regions are not compatible with 1992 data.

8 Casualty rates per 100 million vehicle kilometres: by road class, region[1] and severity: 1990-1992 average

Rate per 100 million vehicle kilometres

	Motorways	A roads Built up Trunk	A roads Built up Principal	A roads Non built up Trunk	A roads Non built up Principal	All A roads	All main roads
Northern[2]							
Fatal	0.6	0.7	1.4	1.3	1.5	1.4	1.3
Fatal & serious	2.4	11.7	17.0	7.2	10.5	11.3	10.3
All severities	17.4	101.2	112.0	37.1	52.2	65.5	60.1
Yorkshire and Humberside							
Fatal	0.4	2.2	1.4	1.2	2.2	1.6	1.3
Fatal & serious	3.0	19.2	19.2	11.1	18.9	16.8	13.3
All severities	15.4	105.1	109.8	39.0	67.3	78.2	62.6
East Midlands							
Fatal	0.4	1.6	1.5	1.6	2.1	1.7	1.5
Fatal & serious	3.7	18.9	18.4	9.8	16.9	14.7	12.6
All severities	19.7	109.9	120.4	41.7	69.2	73.8	63.5
Eastern							
Fatal	0.4	1.5	1.0	1.0	1.6	1.2	1.0
Fatal & serious	2.8	17.7	16.3	7.5	12.9	11.7	9.3
All severities	17.8	98.6	103.4	32.7	57.2	59.2	48.3
South East							
Fatal	0.4	1.3	0.9	0.8	1.4	1.1	0.9
Fatal & serious	2.7	16.3	15.0	5.8	11.9	11.2	8.7
All severities	16.0	99.5	99.4	29.2	56.4	63.0	49.0
London							
Fatal	0.3	1.9	1.7	0.6	0.8	1.5	1.4
Fatal & serious	6.0	24.9	37.1	7.3	11.1	29.4	27.7
All severities	48.0	156.4	223.5	39.0	58.0	177.0	168.1
South West							
Fatal	0.3	0.9	1.1	1.0	1.6	1.3	1.1
Fatal & serious	2.3	12.9	12.8	7.1	12.7	11.2	9.3
All severities	12.2	84.6	73.5	30.0	53.1	53.2	44.8
West Midlands							
Fatal	0.3	1.5	1.5	1.2	1.6	1.4	1.1
Fatal & serious	2.4	14.8	19.1	10.7	13.0	15.1	10.8
All severities	14.6	86.1	109.1	45.1	57.7	78.1	56.5
North West[2]							
Fatal	0.4	2.2	1.6	1.6	1.5	1.6	1.2
Fatal & serious	2.6	16.9	16.7	9.4	11.4	14.2	10.2
All severities	19.7	137.5	139.9	50.8	60.3	105.5	75.8
England							
Fatal	0.4	1.7	1.3	1.1	1.6	1.4	1.1
Fatal & serious	2.8	19.7	20.1	8.1	13.3	14.6	11.6
All severities	17.3	123.0	129.1	36.3	58.4	81.3	65.2
Wales							
Fatal	0.3	1.3	1.4	1.4	1.6	1.5	1.2
Fatal & serious	2.5	15.3	16.3	12.7	15.1	14.5	12.1
All severities	16.9	90.6	112.4	51.3	66.5	74.9	62.7
Scotland							
Fatal	0.5	1.5	1.5	1.9	1.7	1.7	1.5
Fatal & serious	3.2	22.1	23.2	13.7	15.9	17.3	15.2
All severities	15.2	97.1	108.8	44.2	56.3	67.3	59.5
Great Britain							
Fatal	0.4	1.7	1.4	1.2	1.6	1.4	1.2
Fatal & serious	2.8	19.6	20.2	9.1	13.7	14.9	12.0
All severities	17.2	118.7	126.9	38.2	58.6	79.6	64.8

1 Traffic data and casualty data in this breakdown are not available for Northern Ireland.
2 From 1st April 1991 responsibilty for Cumbria transferred from the North West Regional Office to the Northern Regional Office. The change to the road accident database was deferred until 1992.

9 Accident rates per 100 million vehicle kilometres: by road class, region[1] and severity: 1990-1992 average

Rate per 100 million vehicle kilometres

		A roads				All A roads	All main roads
		Built up		Non built up			
	Motorways	Trunk	Principal	Trunk	Principal		
Northern[2]							
Fatal	0.5	0.7	1.4	1.1	1.3	1.3	1.2
Fatal & serious	1.8	11.3	15.6	5.1	7.8	9.2	8.4
All severities	11.3	72.9	85.9	22.2	32.4	45.4	41.5
Yorkshire and Humberside							
Fatal	0.3	1.9	1.3	1.0	1.9	1.4	1.1
Fatal & serious	2.1	16.0	17.1	7.9	13.1	13.3	10.6
All severities	9.6	80.6	85.6	23.2	40.6	55.7	44.3
East Midlands							
Fatal	0.4	1.4	1.5	1.3	1.8	1.5	1.3
Fatal & serious	2.4	16.3	16.6	7.1	11.9	11.5	9.8
All severities	11.4	83.3	94.1	25.3	42.3	51.0	43.4
Eastern							
Fatal	0.3	1.4	1.0	0.8	1.4	1.1	0.9
Fatal & serious	2.0	15.2	14.8	5.5	9.5	9.3	7.4
All severities	11.3	77.4	81.6	20.2	36.1	41.4	33.5
South East							
Fatal	0.3	1.2	0.9	0.7	1.2	1.0	0.8
Fatal & serious	2.0	13.7	13.8	4.3	9.1	9.3	7.1
All severities	9.9	76.1	80.0	18.4	37.1	46.1	35.4
London							
Fatal	0.3	1.8	1.6	0.5	0.8	1.5	1.4
Fatal & serious	4.5	22.1	34.3	6.2	9.0	26.9	25.3
All severities	34.1	127.2	190.9	27.9	42.0	149.0	141.0
South West							
Fatal	0.3	0.9	1.0	0.9	1.3	1.1	0.9
Fatal & serious	1.6	11.1	11.5	5.1	9.4	8.8	7.3
All severities	7.6	65.0	59.4	18.3	33.5	37.4	31.3
West Midlands							
Fatal	0.2	1.5	1.4	1.0	1.4	1.3	0.9
Fatal & serious	1.7	12.6	16.8	7.7	9.8	12.4	8.8
All severities	8.7	63.8	84.0	28.9	36.8	56.5	40.3
North West[2]							
Fatal	0.3	2.0	1.5	1.3	1.4	1.5	1.1
Fatal & serious	1.9	14.5	15.2	6.9	8.4	12.1	8.6
All severities	12.1	98.9	104.1	30.5	38.0	75.5	53.6
England							
Fatal	0.3	1.6	1.3	0.9	1.4	1.2	1.0
Fatal & serious	2.0	17.2	18.3	5.9	9.8	12.2	9.6
All severities	10.8	96.1	103.1	22.6	36.9	60.1	47.7
Wales							
Fatal	0.2	1.2	1.3	1.2	1.5	1.3	1.1
Fatal & serious	1.8	13.1	14.0	8.7	10.7	11.0	9.1
All severities	10.4	67.6	83.4	29.5	40.8	50.0	41.7
Scotland							
Fatal	0.4	1.5	1.4	1.6	1.5	1.5	1.3
Fatal & serious	2.6	19.2	21.2	9.4	11.7	13.7	12.0
All severities	9.8	73.7	87.7	25.8	35.2	47.2	41.6
Great Britain							
Fatal	0.3	1.6	1.3	1.0	1.4	1.3	1.0
Fatal & serious	2.0	17.0	18.3	6.5	10.0	12.3	9.8
All severities	10.7	92.4	101.2	23.4	36.9	58.4	47.0

1 Traffic data and casualty data in this breakdown are not available for Northern Ireland.

2 From 1st April 1991 responsibilty for Cumbria transferred from the North West Regional Office to the Northern Regional Office. The change to the road accident database was deferred until 1992.

10 Accident indices[1]: by month, severity and region: accidents by severity and region: 1992

	Jan	Feb	Mar	Apr	May	Jun	Jul	Aug	Sep	Oct	Nov	Dec	All accidents
Northern[2]													
Fatal & serious	89	93	97	100	97	91	111	93	110	103	113	103	2,134
All	93	95	90	100	97	94	103	101	110	104	113	102	10,510
Yorkshire and Humberside													
Fatal & serious	93	91	92	98	102	104	96	102	97	105	108	113	4,231
All	101	92	90	95	93	99	99	103	107	102	119	102	19,714
East Midlands													
Fatal & serious	95	84	88	106	102	116	103	109	99	88	115	95	3,388
All	100	84	92	95	95	104	105	100	102	103	112	105	16,051
Eastern													
Fatal & serious	104	76	90	94	95	98	105	103	107	105	113	108	5,054
All	100	85	95	93	100	102	100	95	102	101	116	110	24,208
South East													
Fatal & serious	106	89	94	91	97	99	109	99	96	104	107	110	5,415
All	99	87	94	91	101	100	103	98	102	103	113	108	29,152
London													
Fatal & serious	92	93	98	99	109	109	96	91	100	105	109	99	6,575
All	93	92	102	96	99	106	101	93	104	103	112	99	38,748
South West													
Fatal & serious	90	86	92	92	109	101	109	109	103	104	104	100	3,425
All	88	89	87	87	99	106	105	111	103	103	120	103	16,380
West Midlands													
Fatal & serious	93	92	91	98	110	92	102	100	104	94	125	98	4,137
All	93	90	95	98	99	98	105	95	100	103	120	104	20,130
North West[2]													
Fatal & serious	93	91	91	102	98	106	110	99	94	101	117	98	4,250
All	92	92	99	97	100	98	97	98	96	108	115	108	29,648
England													
Fatal & serious	96	88	93	97	102	102	104	100	100	101	112	103	38,609
All	95	89	95	95	99	101	102	98	102	103	115	105	204,541
Wales													
Fatal & serious	84	88	95	99	121	101	120	114	90	88	98	100	2,033
All	90	88	88	98	110	100	107	112	100	98	109	99	10,467
Scotland													
Fatal & serious	103	100	89	91	108	91	96	110	100	102	108	103	4,696
All	98	98	98	95	101	92	99	110	101	102	107	99	18,017
Great Britain													
Fatal & serious	96	89	92	97	104	101	104	102	100	101	111	103	45,338
All	95	90	95	95	99	100	102	100	102	103	114	104	233,025
Northern Ireland													
Fatal & serious	101	95	79	115	105	102	91	101	105	110	102	95	1,453
All	96	94	96	101	97	94	87	100	106	113	117	99	6,650
United Kingdom													
Fatal & serious	96	89	92	97	104	101	103	102	100	101	111	103	46,791
All	95	90	95	95	99	100	101	100	102	103	114	104	239,675

1 The base(=100) is the average number of accidents per day for the region.
2 From 1st April 1991 responsibilty for Cumbria transferred from the North West Regional Office to the Northern Regional Office. The change to the road accident database was deferred until 1992. Consequently data prior to 1992 for both Northern and North West regions are not compatible with 1992 data.

11 Accidents on motorways: by carriageway type, junction, number of lanes, region[1] and severity: 1992

Number of accidents

	Junction			Non−junction		
	Number of lanes		Circular section of roundabouts	Number of lanes		Total[2]
	2	3+		2	3+	
Northern[3]						
Fatal or serious	0	3	1	8	21	34
All severities	27	11	14	45	76	178
Yorkshire and Humberside						
Fatal or serious	6	6	6	10	67	98
All severities	34	20	58	76	296	514
East Midlands						
Fatal or serious	1	5	2	4	60	73
All severities	9	29	12	10	280	361
Eastern						
Fatal or serious	3	13	3	14	122	165
All severities	34	67	9	89	692	967
South East						
Fatal or serious	6	14	8	33	137	223
All severities	59	76	48	161	791	1,281
London						
Fatal or serious	5	10	0	9	35	61
All severities	39	95	6	57	273	482
of which:						
Inner London						
Fatal or serious	2	3	0	1	2	9
All severities	11	22	6	4	14	60
Outer London						
Fatal or serious	3	7	0	8	33	52
All severities	28	73	0	53	259	422
South West						
Fatal or serious	1	3	1	6	59	77
All severities	14	15	14	38	248	370
West Midlands						
Fatal or serious	3	16	0	18	100	147
All severities	15	58	7	80	509	719
North West[3]						
Fatal or serious	4	12	3	12	115	158
All severities	50	68	71	135	787	1,235
England						
Fatal or serious	29	82	24	114	716	1,036
All severities	281	439	239	691	3,952	6,107
Wales						
Fatal or serious	1	0	1	8	16	28
All severities	11	7	9	52	78	162
Scotland						
Fatal or serious	6	5	1	42	30	85
All severities	28	29	4	142	134	361
Great Britain						
Fatal or serious	36	87	26	164	762	1,149
All severities	320	475	252	885	4,164	6,630

1 Accident data are not available in this breakdown for Northern Ireland.
2 Includes unknown carriageway type and slip roads.
3 From 1st April 1991 responsibilty for Cumbria transferred from the North West Regional Office to the Northern Regional Office.
  The change to the road accident database was deferred until 1992. Consequently data prior to 1992 for both Northern and North West regions are not compatible with 1992 data.

12 Accidents on trunk 'A' roads: by carriageway type, junction, number of lanes, region[1] and severity: 1992

Number of accidents

	Dual carriageway					Single carriageway							Circular section of round-about[5]	All trunk A roads[6]
	Junction		Non-junction			Junction			Non-junction					
	Number of lanes[2]		Number of lanes[2]			Number of lanes[3]			Number of lanes[3]					
	2	3+	2	3+	All	2[4]	3	4+	2[4]	3	4+	All		
Northern[7]														
Fatal or serious	28	1	39	2	70	51	4	0	107	3	0	165	10	245
All severities	147	9	230	22	408	244	13	4	298	7	0	566	84	1,062
Yorkshire and Humberside														
Fatal or serious	61	4	81	4	150	99	8	4	132	4	1	248	18	419
All severities	187	9	280	17	493	406	26	26	343	18	10	829	146	1,478
East Midlands														
Fatal or serious	51	5	96	5	157	130	5	2	176	5	3	321	30	508
All severities	219	20	338	7	584	588	29	25	569	12	6	1,229	244	2,061
Eastern														
Fatal or serious	78	10	136	13	237	140	9	2	143	5	0	299	23	563
All severities	327	39	532	68	966	597	27	15	521	18	4	1,182	253	2,411
South East														
Fatal or serious	57	13	93	30	193	81	1	1	112	5	4	204	26	426
All severities	256	76	397	137	866	411	24	8	425	23	6	897	263	2,053
London														
Fatal or serious	107	156	70	105	438	117	5	65	55	3	29	274	31	745
All severities	659	775	353	485	2,272	944	56	422	263	22	109	1,816	299	4,406
of which:														
Inner London														
Fatal or serious	29	49	17	31	126	68	2	48	24	2	16	160	1	287
All severities	199	225	81	106	611	521	27	324	141	5	70	1,088	31	1,735
Outer London														
Fatal or serious	78	107	53	74	312	49	3	17	31	1	13	114	30	458
All severities	460	550	272	379	1,661	423	29	98	122	17	39	728	268	2,671
South West														
Fatal or serious	28	0	54	2	84	75	5	1	90	7	0	178	13	276
All severities	112	2	192	9	315	365	25	7	376	36	1	810	170	1,303
West Midlands														
Fatal or serious	53	7	48	2	110	97	11	0	125	4	0	237	29	377
All severities	215	25	219	10	469	456	30	5	407	8	0	906	222	1,601
North West[7]														
Fatal or serious	22	15	17	4	58	56	5	10	52	3	6	132	15	206
All severities	195	129	127	44	495	369	26	97	214	7	33	746	186	1,439
England														
Fatal or serious	485	211	634	167	1,497	846	53	85	992	39	43	2,058	195	3,765
All severities	2,317	1,084	2,668	799	6,868	4,380	256	609	3,416	151	169	8,981	1,867	17,814
Wales														
Fatal or serious	26	0	48	1	75	88	14	0	185	12	0	299	11	385
All severities	128	9	218	12	367	381	33	1	553	38	1	1,007	96	1,475
Scotland														
Fatal or serious	76	6	106	4	192	147	4	2	347	4	6	510	13	718
All severities	212	28	301	25	566	512	14	16	929	8	22	1,501	66	2,142
Great Britain														
Fatal or serious	587	217	788	172	1,764	1,081	71	87	1,524	55	49	2,867	219	4,868
All severities	2,657	1,121	3,187	836	7,801	5,273	303	626	4,898	197	192	11,489	2,029	21,431

1 Accident data in this breakdown are not available for Northern Ireland.
2 Number of lanes in each direction.
3 Number of lanes in both directions.
4 Includes one way streets.
5 These are classified as junction accidents.
6 Includes unknown carriageway type and single track roads.
7 From 1st April 1991 responsibilty for Cumbria transferred from the North West Regional Office to the Northern Regional Office. The change to the road accident database was deferred until 1992. Consequently data prior to 1992 for both Northern and North West regions are not compatible with 1992 data.

13 Accidents on principal 'A' roads: by carriageway type, junction, number of lanes, region[1] and severity: 1992

Number of accidents

	Dual carriageway					Single carriageway							Circular section of roundabout[5]	All principal A roads[6]
	Junction		Non-junction			Junction			Non-junction					
	Number of lanes[2]		Number of lanes[2]			Number of lanes[3]			Number of lanes[3]					
	2	3+	2	3+	All	2^4	3	4+	2^4	3	4+	All		
Northern[7]														
Fatal or serious	61	9	56	6	132	218	11	18	232	6	12	497	31	669
All severities	282	27	232	34	575	1,264	69	111	907	30	48	2,429	316	3,368
Yorkshire and Humberside														
Fatal or serious	141	22	100	15	278	555	45	28	517	14	9	1,168	65	1,514
All severities	735	179	377	74	1,365	2,703	210	178	1,712	52	43	4,898	502	6,814
East Midlands														
Fatal or serious	61	15	68	4	148	417	12	48	471	7	12	967	49	1,164
All severities	359	94	252	15	720	2,290	101	211	1,699	23	40	4,364	388	5,493
Eastern														
Fatal or serious	81	4	81	5	171	583	36	14	601	21	4	1,259	108	1,541
All severities	505	63	367	29	964	3,192	189	86	2,115	87	17	5,686	923	7,629
South East														
Fatal or serious	154	33	138	15	340	772	43	26	717	21	12	1,591	114	2,062
All severities	869	153	579	65	1,666	4,579	221	200	2,941	73	53	8,067	1,098	11,017
London														
Fatal or serious	351	38	129	17	535	1,601	50	267	583	11	81	2,593	81	3,220
All severities	2,321	292	681	79	3,373	9,868	302	1,579	2,894	60	428	15,131	604	19,175
of which:														
Inner London														
Fatal or serious	202	31	62	10	305	743	33	176	249	10	56	1,267	29	1,606
All severities	1,436	213	374	57	2,080	4,891	184	1,047	1,274	41	301	7,738	234	10,087
Outer London														
Fatal or serious	149	7	67	7	230	858	17	91	334	1	25	1,326	52	1,614
All severities	885	79	307	22	1,293	4,977	118	532	1,620	19	127	7,393	370	9,088
South West														
Fatal or serious	70	9	76	8	163	456	28	10	530	11	6	1,041	64	1,275
All severities	337	36	265	28	666	2,386	121	51	1,935	47	21	4,561	531	5,824
West Midlands														
Fatal or serious	153	46	128	14	341	471	33	63	432	11	21	1,031	81	1,462
All severities	765	218	446	70	1,499	2,764	150	338	1,644	53	99	5,048	596	7,196
North West[7]														
Fatal or serious	152	89	77	46	364	674	28	117	442	9	42	1,312	35	1,729
All severities	1,233	628	481	191	2,533	5,262	254	852	2,038	39	203	8,648	524	11,906
England														
Fatal or serious	1,224	265	853	130	2,472	5,747	286	591	4,525	111	199	11,459	628	14,636
All severities	7,406	1,690	3,680	585	13,361	34,308	1,617	3,606	17,885	464	952	58,832	5,482	78,422
Wales														
Fatal or serious	36	4	26	5	71	213	17	14	331	8	4	587	17	676
All severities	197	25	142	11	375	1,244	87	73	1,247	27	27	2,705	210	3,308
Scotland														
Fatal or serious	92	17	103	17	229	496	20	50	711	6	33	1,316	26	1,597
All severities	404	105	420	66	995	2,022	74	286	2,253	17	128	4,780	233	6,073
Great Britain														
Fatal or serious	1,352	286	982	152	2,772	6,456	323	655	5,567	125	236	13,362	671	16,909
All severities	8,007	1,820	4,242	662	14,731	37,574	1,778	3,965	21,385	508	1,107	66,317	5,925	87,803

1 Accident data in this breakdown are not available for Northern Ireland.
2 Number of lanes in each direction.
3 Number of lanes in both directions.
4 Includes one way streets.
5 These are classified as junction accidents.
6 Includes unknown carriageway type and single track roads.
7 From 1st April 1991 responsibilty for Cumbria transferred from the North West Regional Office to the Northern Regional Office. The change to the road accident database was deferred until 1992. Consequently data prior to 1992 for both Northern and North West regions are not compatible with 1992 data.

35

14 Accidents: by road class, severity, region and county: 1981-85 average, 1991, 1992

Number

	Motorways			Trunk A roads			Principal A roads			All roads		
	Fatal	Fatal or serious	All severities	Fatal	Fatal or serious	All severities	Fatal	Fatal or serious	All severities	Fatal	Fatal or serious	All severities
Northern Region[1]												
1981-85	7	37	118	34	259	833	104	1,009	3,602	260	2,930	10,613
1991	10	36	181	51	247	1,077	94	724	3,536	263	2,241	10,845
1992	8	34	178	47	245	1,062	67	669	3,368	202	2,134	10,510
Cleveland[2]												
1981-85	0	0	0	4	19	97	18	174	770	42	423	2,137
1991	0	0	0	4	14	124	15	121	782	40	320	2,144
1992	0	0	0	1	13	97	12	119	710	24	338	1,996
Cumbria[1]												
1981-85	5	22	62	13	127	355	16	195	605	55	675	2,043
1991	4	23	77	26	115	407	23	135	547	66	472	1,863
1992	5	22	83	21	107	367	14	128	516	59	452	1,780
Durham												
1981-85	2	10	35	7	40	110	24	195	585	55	577	1,801
1991	4	10	66	5	25	170	17	112	519	50	365	1,964
1992	1	6	60	5	39	179	16	106	586	40	360	2,041
Northumberland[2]												
1981-85	0	0	0	7	45	163	11	87	280	35	313	1,043
1991	0	0	0	10	57	203	10	86	386	35	265	1,132
1992	0	0	0	13	56	201	12	68	312	31	224	1,008
Tyne and Wear												
1981-85	0	5	21	2	29	107	36	357	1,361	73	942	3,588
1991	2	3	38	6	36	173	29	270	1,302	72	819	3,742
1992	2	6	35	7	30	218	13	248	1,244	48	760	3,685
Yorkshire and Humberside Region												
1981-85	14	78	306	65	541	1,498	196	2,053	6,932	463	5,714	20,018
1991	18	116	500	61	432	1,472	145	1,536	6,763	367	4,352	19,699
1992	17	98	514	43	419	1,478	158	1,514	6,814	373	4,231	19,714
Humberside												
1981-85	2	10	33	8	72	243	28	308	1,201	73	996	3,894
1991	2	8	45	8	50	210	25	232	1,083	64	809	3,755
1992	5	15	58	5	59	226	30	253	1,074	78	850	3,872
North Yorkshire												
1981-85	0	3	8	24	239	467	29	474	1,048	82	1,423	3,128
1991	0	3	11	24	198	553	28	374	1,064	79	1,051	3,166
1992	1	5	8	16	194	493	24	351	1,043	71	1,013	3,048
South Yorkshire												
1981-85	4	26	110	10	75	250	42	420	1,654	103	1,123	4,631
1991	7	42	186	10	46	214	30	281	1,515	88	774	4,330
1992	5	31	183	10	53	246	39	279	1,557	86	721	4,407
West Yorkshire												
1981-85	7	39	155	23	155	538	96	851	3,030	205	2,172	8,365
1991	9	63	258	19	138	495	62	649	3,101	136	1,718	8,448
1992	6	47	265	12	113	513	65	631	3,140	138	1,647	8,387
East Midlands Region												
1981-85	15	129	390	97	792	2,350	158	1,770	5,721	443	5,334	17,379
1991	13	95	424	77	519	2,106	143	1,182	5,597	366	3,451	16,376
1992	16	73	361	88	508	2,061	119	1,164	5,493	346	3,388	16,051
Derbyshire												
1981-85	2	18	69	20	159	545	34	339	1,130	97	1,057	3,743
1991	4	16	88	11	94	544	20	141	1,104	63	488	3,485
1992	5	18	91	20	129	563	17	155	1,090	69	545	3,551
Leicestershire												
1981-85	6	24	93	16	115	360	32	330	1,198	93	1,042	3,702
1991	7	33	130	15	78	313	28	212	1,157	82	631	3,456
1992	8	22	124	15	68	275	27	189	1,216	81	593	3,453

1 From 1st April 1991 responsibilty for Cumbria transferred from the North West Regional Office to the Northern Regional Office.
  The change to the road accident database was deferred until 1992. However, for this table data prior to 1992 have been changed to take account of the new boundaries.
2 This county contains no motorways.

Number

	Motorways			Trunk A roads			Principal A roads			All roads		
	Fatal	Fatal or serious	All severities	Fatal	Fatal or serious	All severities	Fatal	Fatal or serious	All severities	Fatal	Fatal or serious	All severities
Lincolnshire[1]												
1981-85	0	0	0	20	160	454	29	294	932	76	852	2,683
1991	0	0	0	16	109	328	28	258	895	65	620	2,315
1992	0	0	0	18	81	327	30	260	913	62	624	2,440
Northamptonshire												
1981-85	6	75	190	18	182	434	22	381	1,011	69	1,025	2,673
1991	2	36	152	13	93	316	25	226	940	53	647	2,380
1992	2	22	101	16	90	306	26	225	854	58	587	2,227
Nottinghamshire												
1981-85	1	11	38	22	175	557	41	426	1,450	108	1,359	4,577
1991	0	10	54	22	145	605	42	345	1,501	103	1,065	4,740
1992	1	11	45	19	140	590	19	335	1,420	76	1,039	4,380
Eastern Region												
1981-85	20	153	560	104	876	2,591	199	2,488	8,215	543	7,727	25,186
1991	25	180	951	101	642	2,538	177	1,626	7,556	486	5,168	24,513
1992	22	165	967	66	563	2,411	175	1,541	7,629	434	5,054	24,208
Bedfordshire												
1981-85	4	29	109	10	94	345	17	160	622	50	600	2,444
1991	4	22	107	10	50	293	20	104	536	53	385	2,060
1992	5	22	113	8	52	297	17	96	544	45	375	2,111
Buckinghamshire												
1981-85	5	38	120	3	36	110	27	318	1,001	63	843	2,617
1991	5	32	226	9	21	105	16	131	883	44	366	2,588
1992	8	26	201	3	13	110	26	139	911	59	402	2,744
Cambridgeshire												
1981-85	1	5	19	23	158	462	25	303	1,009	75	908	2,979
1991	1	5	33	19	141	527	28	293	1,119	74	853	3,516
1992	1	2	22	13	127	522	30	262	1,149	63	797	3,389
Essex												
1981-85	3	29	109	11	97	321	53	675	2,398	125	2,032	6,976
1991	9	45	246	19	80	453	31	337	2,105	98	1,095	6,677
1992	2	39	225	13	82	403	30	351	2,037	83	1,132	6,322
Hertfordshire												
1981-85	7	53	203	16	121	404	30	393	1,469	84	1,177	4,316
1991	6	76	339	10	83	291	37	280	1,177	83	930	3,881
1992	6	76	406	7	73	305	22	251	1,162	57	898	3,991
Norfolk[1]												
1981-85	0	0	0	21	190	461	27	360	910	82	1,207	3,110
1991	0	0	0	20	164	532	33	271	990	84	914	3,430
1992	0	0	0	14	123	415	36	253	1,084	95	884	3,387
Suffolk[1]												
1981-85	0	0	0	20	179	488	19	280	805	64	960	2,744
1991	0	0	0	14	103	337	12	210	746	50	625	2,361
1992	0	0	0	8	93	359	14	189	742	32	566	2,264
South East Region												
1981-85	29	205	652	109	800	2,453	282	3,500	12,091	677	9,327	32,192
1991	29	215	1,126	66	424	2,105	197	2,058	10,628	478	5,477	28,850
1992	40	223	1,281	55	426	2,053	184	2,062	11,017	463	5,415	29,152
Berkshire												
1981-85	10	69	215	7	61	195	24	321	1,167	71	942	3,263
1991	8	38	220	7	18	152	12	123	951	37	372	2,737
1992	7	39	241	1	10	95	10	135	1,081	41	359	2,816
East Sussex[1]												
1981-85	0	0	0	10	78	232	31	347	1,163	66	838	2,997
1991	0	0	0	6	38	165	25	240	1,068	50	535	2,727
1992	0	0	0	5	44	198	21	196	1,082	49	482	2,742

1 This county contains no motorways.

Number

	Motorways			Trunk A roads			Principal A roads			All roads		
	Fatal	Fatal or serious	All severities	Fatal	Fatal or serious	All severities	Fatal	Fatal or serious	All severities	Fatal	Fatal or serious	All severities
Hampshire												
1981-85	4	36	109	21	160	437	50	792	2,416	140	2,320	7,227
1991	2	43	187	9	77	357	37	451	2,129	99	1,391	6,715
1992	3	45	208	5	64	273	37	482	2,184	96	1,385	6,643
Isle of Wight[1]												
1981-85	0	0	0	0	0	0	4	70	214	8	155	495
1991	0	0	0	0	0	0	1	40	171	5	95	400
1992	0	0	0	0	0	0	3	54	180	5	115	421
Kent												
1981-85	7	49	162	21	175	539	63	779	2,543	142	2,053	6,819
1991	9	39	218	9	113	554	57	470	2,242	117	1,220	5,950
1992	12	49	248	21	150	606	49	473	2,341	114	1,331	6,185
Oxfordshire												
1981-85	1	6	12	24	164	521	26	279	801	71	871	2,531
1991	3	15	83	20	71	331	17	126	799	61	368	2,232
1992	6	20	91	11	65	359	23	158	821	53	408	2,303
Surrey												
1981-85	7	43	144	10	62	224	52	613	2,618	109	1,391	5,870
1991	7	76	397	5	36	232	26	381	2,209	62	934	5,295
1992	11	67	471	7	44	251	24	355	2,249	64	858	5,297
West Sussex												
1981-85	0	2	9	16	102	306	31	299	1,170	70	757	2,990
1991	0	4	21	10	71	314	22	227	1,059	47	562	2,794
1992	1	3	22	5	49	271	17	209	1,079	41	477	2,745
London												
1981-85	6	35	266	56	413	2,489	301	4,269	25,584	521	7,588	45,274
1991	3	55	435	59	834	4,588	184	3,506	19,272	349	7,267	39,454
1992	3	61	482	62	745	4,406	135	3,220	19,175	308	6,575	38,748
Inner London												
1981-85[2]	..	..	..	..	..	..	..	..	..	212	3,383	20,946
1991	1	5	62	21	301	1,768	81	1,832	10,214	149	3,334	18,460
1992	1	9	60	17	287	1,735	58	1,606	10,087	112	2,949	18,100
Outer London												
1981-85[2]	..	..	..	..	..	..	..	..	..	309	4,204	24,327
1991	2	50	373	38	533	2,820	103	1,674	9,058	200	3,933	20,994
1992	2	52	422	45	458	2,671	77	1,614	9,088	196	3,626	20,648
South West Region												
1981-85	17	127	344	62	585	1,586	197	2,475	7,390	440	6,697	19,847
1991	15	81	405	50	348	1,307	180	1,404	6,066	406	3,793	16,765
1992	13	77	370	55	276	1,303	140	1,275	5,824	335	3,425	16,380
Avon												
1981-85	8	50	124	3	29	61	41	450	1,415	86	1,149	3,596
1991	9	30	168	2	11	48	36	219	979	84	579	2,824
1992	5	23	150	3	16	49	27	170	827	65	480	2,629
Cornwall[1]												
1981-85	0	0	0	10	92	249	14	236	667	39	696	1,984
1991	0	0	0	7	63	237	10	139	602	24	427	1,838
1992	0	0	0	11	50	250	15	127	585	37	368	1,770
Devon												
1981-85	2	10	27	13	131	345	35	570	1,563	82	1,568	4,354
1991	1	11	49	10	102	325	27	282	1,165	76	944	3,768
1992	2	14	51	12	61	298	17	291	1,139	55	863	3,690
Dorset[1]												
1981-85	0	0	0	4	45	148	23	311	1,112	48	803	2,779
1991	0	0	0	7	43	130	27	183	994	52	476	2,403
1992	0	0	0	6	23	148	24	182	1,034	47	428	2,427

1 This county contains no motorways.
2 Trunk road data are not available for these years.

Number

	Motorways			Trunk A roads			Principal A roads			All roads		
	Fatal	Fatal or serious	All severities	Fatal	Fatal or serious	All severities	Fatal	Fatal or serious	All severities	Fatal	Fatal or serious	All severities
Gloucestershire												
1981-85	1	21	54	13	145	369	24	282	705	59	967	2,479
1991	0	13	56	14	56	269	19	162	709	52	425	1,971
1992	2	7	52	9	50	269	11	141	692	43	386	2,051
Somerset												
1981-85	3	17	43	6	48	117	29	295	789	57	666	1,783
1991	2	9	52	3	25	74	33	192	761	65	403	1,724
1992	1	9	46	4	14	60	24	167	710	40	372	1,646
Wiltshire												
1981-85	4	28	96	12	94	297	32	331	1,138	68	847	2,871
1991	3	18	79	7	48	224	28	227	856	53	539	2,237
1992	3	24	71	10	62	229	22	197	837	48	528	2,167
West Midlands Region												
1981-85	19	138	476	81	639	1,827	190	2,263	7,415	484	6,527	21,030
1991	18	133	746	49	384	1,624	151	1,538	7,210	363	4,447	20,565
1992	19	147	719	59	377	1,601	150	1,462	7,196	357	4,137	20,130
Hereford and Worcester												
1981-85	4	29	104	10	83	245	31	329	1,060	71	859	2,762
1991	2	20	130	11	70	279	26	215	959	55	556	2,660
1992	3	24	116	10	63	321	28	197	899	53	509	2,534
Shropshire												
1981-85	0	2	4	14	147	363	17	170	473	51	653	1,611
1991	0	4	14	9	94	307	10	123	406	30	444	1,584
1992	1	1	9	12	85	242	18	132	465	49	406	1,546
Staffordshire												
1981-85	8	36	146	25	163	602	36	405	1,577	105	1,209	4,813
1991	5	27	244	16	89	560	27	254	1,738	66	698	4,958
1992	1	19	208	17	104	582	29	216	1,611	72	632	4,679
Warwickshire												
1981-85	4	29	68	19	148	336	23	220	553	77	850	2,078
1991	5	46	143	7	70	225	10	150	557	52	634	2,192
1992	7	51	171	14	76	236	13	171	616	48	665	2,246
West Midlands												
1981-85	4	41	154	12	98	280	84	1,140	3,752	180	2,956	9,767
1991	6	36	215	6	61	253	78	796	3,550	160	2,115	9,171
1992	7	52	215	6	49	220	62	746	3,605	135	1,925	9,125
North West Region[1]												
1981-85	29	158	749	48	314	1,252	232	2,208	10,622	503	5,504	26,599
1991	29	161	1,044	42	253	1,406	204	1,819	11,798	439	4,442	28,892
1992	37	158	1,235	32	206	1,439	190	1,729	11,906	408	4,250	29,648
Cheshire												
1981-85	8	44	198	17	92	400	32	277	1,436	83	778	3,913
1991	8	51	292	17	77	412	32	230	1,453	84	593	3,919
1992	9	45	343	10	49	388	29	212	1,459	73	540	3,951
Greater Manchester												
1981-85	10	59	337	6	50	214	90	971	4,966	178	2,149	11,127
1991	13	53	478	3	39	219	95	799	5,458	164	1,760	12,239
1992	16	58	543	2	24	233	82	720	5,462	153	1,613	12,510
Lancashire												
1981-85	8	40	147	17	113	377	60	554	2,161	135	1,478	5,803
1991	8	40	164	15	80	386	35	388	2,218	102	1,076	5,823
1992	7	39	207	15	95	447	46	412	2,212	109	1,133	6,058
Merseyside												
1981-85	3	14	67	7	59	260	50	406	2,059	107	1,099	5,756
1991	0	17	110	7	57	389	42	402	2,669	89	1,013	6,911
1992	5	16	142	5	38	371	33	385	2,773	73	964	7,129

1 From 1st April 1991 responsibilty for Cumbria transferred from the North West Regional Office to the Northern Regional Office.
The change to the road accident database was deferred until 1992. However, for this table data prior to 1992 have been changed to take account of the new boundaries.

14 Accidents: by road class, severity, region[1] and county: 1981-85 average, 1991, 1992 (cont.)

Number

	Motorways			Trunk A roads			Principal A roads			All roads		
	Fatal	Fatal or serious	All severities	Fatal	Fatal or serious	All severities	Fatal	Fatal or serious	All severities	Fatal	Fatal or serious	All severities
England												
1981-85	156	1,059	3,860	654	5,220	16,880	1,859	22,035	87,572	4,333	57,347	218,137
1991	160	1,072	5,813	556	4,083	18,223	1,475	15,393	78,426	3,517	40,638	205,959
1992	175	1,036	6,107	507	3,765	17,814	1,318	14,636	78,422	3,226	38,609	204,541
Wales												
1981-85	5	38	124	62	620	1,746	86	984	3,427	233	3,082	10,583
1991	3	26	184	53	442	1,630	77	671	3,484	201	2,112	10,830
1992	3	28	162	54	385	1,475	73	676	3,308	206	2,033	10,467
Scotland												
1981-85	16	110	265	138	1,010	2,433	228	2,751	7,438	581	7,412	20,471
1991	15	89	292	117	799	2,353	153	1,764	6,521	440	5,169	19,009
1992	13	85	361	119	718	2,142	145	1,597	6,073	423	4,696	18,017
Great Britain												
1981-85	177	1,207	4,249	854	6,850	21,058	2,173	25,769	98,436	5,147	67,842	249,192
1991	178	1,187	6,289	726	5,324	22,206	1,705	17,828	88,431	4,158	47,919	235,798
1992	191	1,149	6,630	680	4,868	21,431	1,536	16,909	87,803	3,855	45,338	233,025

1 Accident data are not available in this breakdown for Northern Ireland.

15 Accidents and casualties by severity: vehicles involved by vehicle type: road length: all by selected individual motorways[1]: 1992

	Accidents			Casualties			Vehicles involved				Kilo-metres open at December 1992[3]
	Fatal	Serious	All severities	Fatal	Serious	All severities	Two-wheel motor vehicles	Cars and LGV	HGV	All vehicles[2]	
England											
M1, M10	30	126	867	40	200	1,471	42	1,763	341	2,175	306
M45	1	1	3	1	2	4	0	2	0	3	13
M2	3	13	93	3	17	135	5	154	28	193	43
M3	5	38	189	5	44	287	17	374	38	434	86
M4	11	76	581	15	104	885	36	1,142	103	1,304	188
M5	11	53	315	17	76	510	8	576	70	668	262
M6	29	131	937	36	177	1,623	28	1,804	393	2,262	379
M11	1	14	118	1	18	174	4	180	29	220	85
M18	1	10	56	1	23	93	3	91	20	114	45
M20	6	11	92	6	13	140	5	150	38	196	82
M23	1	14	70	1	17	143	4	199	16	225	27
M25	13	109	764	19	145	1,192	29	1,511	237	1,793	189
M26	1	3	9	1	7	20	0	16	2	18	16
M27, M271, M275	2	13	103	2	20	154	4	208	20	235	86
M40	11	31	228	15	53	409	10	400	51	463	145
M42	3	33	114	3	35	180	5	202	45	261	72
M50	1	1	13	1	1	16	0	13	1	14	35
M53	0	5	44	0	5	58	3	68	5	79	33
M54	1	2	21	2	5	33	1	31	7	40	36
M55	0	4	16	0	9	33	2	28	1	32	20
M56	4	8	128	6	11	188	3	239	19	263	58
M57	2	4	38	2	4	52	0	52	10	62	18
M58	0	1	21	0	1	28	2	29	3	34	19
M61	6	13	83	7	17	132	3	164	39	209	40
M62	12	51	407	14	81	698	10	863	285	1,171	167
M63	1	8	88	1	12	134	2	149	13	168	25
M65	0	2	17	0	3	23	0	30	0	30	13
M66	2	3	38	2	5	67	2	73	12	87	19
M69	0	3	16	0	3	17	0	23	4	27	28
M180 & M181	3	5	30	3	5	54	0	18	7	25	45
Other motorways	3	12	146	3	18	219	9	317	44	373	46
Motorways	164	798	5,645	207	1,131	9,172	237	10,869	1,881	13,178	2,626
A(M) roads	11	63	462	12	83	669	39	823	84	962	159
Total (inc A(M) roads)	175	861	6,107	219	1,214	9,841	276	11,692	1,965	14,140	2,785
Wales											
Motorways	3	24	158	3	31	262	4	285	36	334	116
A(M) roads	0	1	4	0	2	6	0	9	0	9	4
Total (inc A(M) roads)	3	25	162	3	33	268	4	294	36	343	120
Scotland											
Motorways	13	72	360	16	91	512	15	588	87	707	279
A(M) roads	0	0	1	0	0	1	0	1	0	1	6
Total (inc A(M) roads)	13	72	361	16	91	513	15	589	87	708	285
Great Britain											
Motorways	180	894	6,163	226	1,253	9,946	256	11,742	2,004	14,219	3,021
A(M) roads	11	64	467	12	85	676	39	833	84	972	169
Total (inc A(M) roads)	191	958	6,630	238	1,338	10,622	295	12,575	2,088	15,191	3,190

1 Motorway accident data are not available in this breakdown for Northern Ireland.
2 Includes pedal cycles, buses and coaches and other vehicles.
3 Excluding slip roads. Data for England from DoT Highways Computing Division. Data for Wales from Welsh Office and Scotland from Scottish Office.

16 Distribution of accidents by road class and region[1]: 1991, 1992

percentage (row sums = 100)

	Motorways		Trunk roads		Principal roads		Other roads	
	1991	1992	1991	1992	1991	1992	1991	1992
Northern[2]	1.2	1.7	7.5	10.1	33.3	32.0	58.1	56.2
Yorkshire and Humberside	2.5	2.6	7.5	7.5	34.3	34.6	55.7	55.3
East Midlands	2.6	2.2	12.9	12.8	34.2	34.2	50.4	50.7
Eastern	3.9	4.0	10.4	10.0	30.8	31.5	54.9	54.5
South Eastern	3.9	4.4	7.3	7.0	36.8	37.8	52.0	50.8
London	1.1	1.2	11.6	11.4	48.8	49.5	38.4	37.9
South West	2.4	2.3	7.8	8.0	36.2	35.5	53.6	54.2
West Midlands	3.6	3.6	7.9	8.0	35.1	35.7	53.4	52.7
North West[2]	3.6	4.2	5.9	4.9	40.1	40.2	50.3	50.8
England	2.8	3.0	8.8	8.7	38.1	38.3	50.3	50.0
Wales	1.7	1.5	15.1	14.1	32.2	31.6	51.1	52.8
Scotland	1.5	2.0	12.4	11.9	34.3	33.7	51.8	52.4
Great Britain	2.7	2.8	9.4	9.2	37.5	37.7	50.4	50.3

1 Accident data in this breakdown are not available for Northern Ireland.
2 From 1st April 1991 responsibilty for Cumbria transferred from the North West Regional Office to the Northern Regional Office.
The change to the road accident database was deferred until 1992. Consequently, the data prior to 1992 for both the Northern and North West regions are not compatible with 1992 data.

17 Motor vehicles, population, area and road length (motorways and built-up and non built-up roads: by trunk and principal): by region: 1992

Thousands/ number

	Motor vehicles currently licensed[1] (thousands)	Population[2] mid year (home) (thousands)	Area in hectares (thousands)	Road length (kilometres)				
				Motorways[3]	Built-up[4]		Non built-up[4]	
					Trunk	Principal	Trunk	Principal
Northern[5]	1,130	3,092	1,540	168	55	615	749	1,409
Yorkshire and Humberside	2,070	4,983	1,542	315	113	1,160	636	1,386
East Midlands	1,769	4,035	1,563	185	153	775	1,076	1,955
Eastern	3,002	5,789	2,100	316	103	1,106	1,203	2,329
South East	3,508	7,040	1,722	574	99	1,542	853	2,369
London	2,751	6,890	158	58	203	1,350	147	40
South West	2,424	4,718	2,385	299	62	1,118	1,041	2,883
West Midlands	2,497	5,265	1,301	378	126	1,131	749	1,593
North West[5]	2,577	6,396	733	463	99	1,683	402	965
England[6]	21,722	48,208	13,044	2,759	1,013	10,481	6,857	14,927
Wales	1,229	2,891	2,077	120	212	851	1,378	1,791
Scotland	1,900	4,921	7,717	269	211	1,244	2,661	6,403
Great Britain[6]	24,851	56,021	22,838	3,147	1,435	12,576	10,896	23,121
Northern Ireland[7]	578	1,594	1,412	112	494		1,718	
United Kingdom[6] [7]	25,429	57,615	24,250	3,259	14,505		35,735	

1 Includes agricultural tractors, combine harvesters, mowing machines, digging machines, mobile cranes, works trucks, pedestrian controlled vehicles, tricycles, showmen's vehicles, general haulage tractors, public service vehicles and exempt vehicles, which represent 2.8 per cent of the total.
2 Final 1991 population estimates were used for England, Wales and Scotland. Provisional 1991 estimates were used for Northern Ireland.
3 Excluding slip roads. Data for England from DoT Highways Computing Division. Total for England includes figures for non-trunk motorways not included in regional totals. Data for Wales from Welsh Office and Scotland from Scottish Office.
4 As at April 1992. Taken from DoT Transport Statistics Report 'Road lengths in Great Britain 1992'.
5 From 1st April 1991 responsibilty for Cumbria transferred from the North West Regional Office to the Northern Regional Office. Consequently, the data prior to 1992 for both the Northern and North West regions are not compatible with 1992 data.
6 Including region of registration unknown.
7 Trunk and Principal road length data are not available for Northern Ireland. Data are for all A roads.

42

18 Motor traffic distribution between regions[1]: by motorway and built-up and non built-up trunk and principal roads: 1990-1992 average

	Motorways	Built-up		Non built-up		All major roads
		Trunk	Principal	Trunk	Principal	
Northern[3]	2	2	4	5	5	4
Yorkshire & Humberside	8	7	9	8	7	8
East Midlands	6	9	6	10	9	8
Eastern	15	7	8	17	15	13
South East	20	8	13	15	18	16
London	2	32	15	5	0	7
South West	9	5	9	10	14	10
West Midlands	14	9	10	7	8	10
North West[3]	16	7	15	6	7	11
England	92	85	89	82	84	87
Wales	3	7	4	6	5	5
Scotland	5	8	7	12	11	9
Great Britain	100	100	100	100	100	100

percent[2]

1 Traffic data are not available for Northern Ireland.
2 Figures have been rounded to the nearest whole number.
3 From 1st April 1991 responsibilty for Cumbria transferred from the North West Regional Office to the Northern Regional Office. The change to the road accident database was deferred until 1992.

19 Motor traffic distribution between motorways, built-up and non built-up trunk and principal roads: by region[1]: 1990-1992 average

	Motorways	Built-up		Non built-up		All major roads
		Trunk	Principal	Trunk	Principal	
Northern[3]	11	1	26	30	31	100
Yorkshire & Humberside	25	3	31	22	19	100
East Midlands	19	5	20	30	26	100
Eastern	26	2	17	30	25	100
South East	30	2	22	21	25	100
London	7	17	58	16	1	100
South West	21	2	23	23	32	100
West Midlands	34	4	28	16	18	100
North West[3]	35	2	36	12	15	100
England	25	4	28	22	22	100
Wales	14	5	22	30	24	100
Scotland	15	3	23	32	28	100
Great Britain	24	4	27	23	22	100

percent[2]

1 Traffic data are not available for Northern Ireland.
2 Figures have been rounded to the nearest whole number.
3 From 1st April 1991 responsibilty for Cumbria transferred from the North West Regional Office to the Northern Regional Office. The change to the road accident database was deferred until 1992.

Definitions

Accident: One involving personal injury occurring on the public highway (including footways) in which a road vehicle is involved and which becomes known to the police within 30 days of its occurrence. The vehicle need not be moving and it need not be in collision with anything. One accident may give rise to several *casualties*. Damage-only accidents are not included in this publication.

'A' Roads: All purpose *trunk* roads and *principal* local authority roads.

Adults: Persons aged 16 years and over.

Built-up Roads: Roads with speed limits (ignoring temporary limits) of 40 mph or less. The pre-1982 definition of 'built-up areas' referred to the same roads but the general nature of the area was never relevant. 'Non built-up roads' refer to those with speed limits of over 40 mph. *Motorways* are included with non built-up roads unless otherwise stated. In tables where data for *motorways* are shown separately, the totals for built-up and non built-up roads exclude *motorway accidents*. In comparing such tables with those involving a built-up/non built-up split only, negligible error will be made by assuming that *motorway accidents* were all on non built-up roads.

Cars: Includes taxis, estate cars, invalid tricycles, three and four-wheeled cars, minibuses and motor caravans.

Casualty: A person *killed* or injured in an *accident*. Casualties are classified as either *killed*, *seriously injured* or *slightly injured*.

Children: Persons under 16 years of age.

Fatal Accident: One in which at least one person is *killed* (but excluding confirmed suicides).

Goods Vehicles: These are divided into two groups according to vehicle weight. They include three-wheeled goods vehicles (eg milk floats) provided they are not controlled by a pedestrian, tankers, tractor units travelling without their semi-trailers, trailers and articulated vehicles.

> *Heavy goods vehicles (HGV):* Those over 1.524 tonnes unladen weight. Includes vehicles with six or more tyres and some four-wheel vehicles with extra large bodies and larger rear tyres. Includes a tractor unit travelling without its usual trailer.

> *Light goods vehicles (LGV):* Vehicles not over 1.524 tonnes unladen weight. Light vans mainly include vehicles of the van type constructed on a car chassis.

Killed: Human *casualties* who sustained injuries resulting in death within 30 days of the *accident*.

KSI: Killed and seriously injured.

Licensed Vehicles: The stock of vehicles currently licensed on 31 December, when the annual census is taken at the Driver and Vehicle Licensing Agency (DVLA).

London: Where possible, data for London have been split into Inner and Outer London. Inner London comprises the City of London and the boroughs of Westminster, Camden, Islington, Hackney, Tower Hamlets, Lewisham, Southwark, Lambeth, Wandsworth, Hammersmith, Kensington and Chelsea, Newham and Haringey. Outer London is all other London boroughs, and includes Heathrow Airport. This definition conforms to that used by the Office of Population Censuses and Surveys (OPCS). See also *Regions*.

Major Roads: These are *motorways*, A(M) and *A class roads* (both *trunk* and *principal*).

Motorcyclist: Riders and passengers of two-wheeled motor vehicles.

Motorways: Data given for motorways are for both motorways and A(M) roads except where otherwise noted. The motorway lengths given in Tables 15 and 17 are main line lengths and exclude associated slip roads.

Motorway Accident: *Accidents* on *motorways* include those on associated slip roads and those at junctions between *motorways* and other roads where the *accident* cannot be clearly allocated to the other road.

Other Roads: These are 'B' and 'C' class roads and unclassified roads, including 'road class not reported'.

Pedal cycle: Includes tandems, tricycles and toy cycles ridden on the carriageway. Also includes battery-assisted cycles and tricycles with a maximum speed of 15 mph.

Pedal cyclist: Riders of pedal cycles including any passengers.

Pedestrians: Also includes persons riding toy cycles on the footway, persons pushing bicycles or pushing or pulling other vehicles or operating pedestrian-controlled vehicles, those leading or herding animals, occupants of prams or wheelchairs, and persons who alight safely from vehicles and are subsequently injured.

Population: The population data used in calculating rates are the final mid-1991 estimates based on 1991 Census results. Mid-year estimates for 1992 were not available at the time of going to publication. The estimates include residents who are temporarily outside the country, and exclude both foreign visitors and members of HM armed forces who are stationed abroad.

Principal Roads: Roads for which County Councils (Regional and Island Authorities in Scotland) are the Highway Authority. The classified *principal roads* (which include local authority *motorways*) are those of regional and urban strategic importance.

Regions: In tables where data are disaggregated by region, Department of Transport (DOT) regions are used, as illustrated by the map on page 2. Greater London is not strictly a region and special arrangements apply, in that the responsibility falls to the London Regional Office (LRO) in DOT headquarters. The South East and Eastern regions do not include any of the Greater London area.

Serious Accident: One in which at least one person is *seriously injured* but no person (other than a confirmed suicide) is killed.

Serious Injury: An injury for which a person is detained in hospital as an 'in-patient', or any of the following injuries whether or not the *casualty* was detained in hospital: fractures, concussion, internal injuries, crushings, severe cuts and lacerations, severe general shock requiring medical treatment, injuries causing death 30 or more days after the *accident*. An injured *casualty* is coded as seriously or *slightly injured* by the police on the basis of information available within a short time of the *accident*. This generally will not include the result of a medical examination, but may include the fact of being detained in hospital, the reasons for which may vary from area to area.

Severity: Of an *accident,* the severity of the most severely injured *casualty* (either fatal, serious or slight); of a casualty, killed, seriously injured or slightly injured.

Slight Accident: One in which at least one person is *slightly injured*, but no person is *killed* or *seriously injured*.

Slight Injury: An injury of a minor character such as a sprain, bruise or cut which are not judged to be severe, or slight shock requiring roadside attention only.

Two-wheel motor vehicles: Mopeds, motor scooters and motor cycles (including motor cycle combinations.

Trunk Roads: Roads comprising the national network of through routes for which the Secretary of State for Transport in England and the Secretaries of State for Scotland and Wales are the highway authorities. The network contains both *motorways*, which legally are special roads reserved for certain classes of traffic, and all-purpose roads which are open to all classes of traffic.

Accident Record Attendant Circumstances

Department of Transport

Stats 19 (Rev 2/91)

1.1 Record Type
1 2
1 New accident record
5 Amended accident record

1.2 Police Force
3 4

1.3 Accident Ref No
5 6 7 8 9 10 11

1.4 Severity of Accident
12
1 Fatal 2 Serious 3 Slight

1.5 Number of Vehicles
13 14 15

1.6 Number of Casualty Records
16 17 18

1.7 Date
Day 19 20 Month 21 22 Year 23 24

1.8 Day of Week
1 Sunday 2 Monday
3 Tuesday 4 Wednesday
5 Thursday 6 Friday
7 Saturday
25

1.9 Time
Hrs 26 27 Mins 28 29
24 hour

1.10 Local Authority
30 31 32

1.11 Location
10 digit reference No
33 34 35 36 37 Easting
38 39 40 41 42
43 Northing

1.12 1st Road Class
1 Motorway
2 A (M)
3 A
4 B
5 C
6 Unclassified
7 Local
8 Authority
9 Use Only

1.13 1st Road Number
44 45 46 47

1.14 Carriageway Type or Markings
48
1 Roundabout (on circular highway)
2 One way street
3 Dual carriageway - 2 lanes
4 Dual carriageway - 3 or more lanes
5 Single carriageway - single track road
6 Single carriageway - 2 lanes (one each direction)
7 Single carriageway - 3 lanes (two way capacity)
8 Single carriageway - 4 or more lanes (two way capacity)
9 Unknown

1.15 Speed Limit
mph
49 50 51
0

1.16 Junction Detail
52 53
0
0 Not at or within 20 metres of junction
1 Roundabout
2 Mini-roundabout
3 'T' or staggered junction
4 'Y' junction
5 Slip road
6 Crossroads
7 Multiple junction
8 Using private drive or entrance
9 Other junction

Junction Accidents Only

1.17 Junction Control
54
1 Authorised person
2 Automatic traffic signal
3 Stop sign
4 Give way sign or markings
5 Uncontrolled

1.18 2nd Road Class
55
1 Motorway
2 A (M)
3 A
4 B
5 C
6 Unclassified
7 Local
8 Authority
9 Use Only

1.19 2nd Road Number
56 57 58 59

1.20 Pedestrian Crossing Facilities
60 61
0
0 No crossing facilities within 50 metres
1 Zebra
2 Zebra crossing controlled by school crossing patrol
3 Zebra crossing controlled by other authorised person
4 Pelican
5 Other light controlled crossing
6 Other sites controlled by school crossing patrol
7 Other sites controlled by other authorised person
8 Central refuge - no other controls
9 Footbridge or subway

1.21 Light Conditions
62
DAYLIGHT
1 Street lights 7 metres or more high
2 Street lights under 7 metres high
3 No street lighting
4 Daylight street lighting unknown
DARKNESS
5 Street lights 7 metres or more high (lit)
6 Street lights under 7 metres high (lit)
7 No street lighting
8 Street lights unlit
9 Darkness street lighting unknown

1.22 Weather
63
1 Fine (without high winds)
2 Raining (without high winds)
3 Snowing (without high winds)
4 Fine with high winds
5 Raining with high winds
6 Snowing with high winds
7 Fog (or mist if hazard)
8 Other
9 Unknown

1.23 Road Surface Condition
64
1 Dry
2 Wet/Damp
3 Snow
4 Frost/Ice
5 Flood (surface water over 3cms (1 inch) deep)

1.24 Special Conditions at Site
65
0 None
1 Automatic Traffic Signal-out
2 Automatic Traffic Signal partially defective
3 Permanent road signing defective or obscured
4 Road works present
5 Road surface defective

1.25 Carriageway Hazards
66
0 None
1 Dislodged vehicle load in carriageway
2 Other object in carriageway
3 Involvement with previous accident
4 Dog in carriageway
5 Other animal in carriageway

1.26 Overtaking Manoeuvre Patterns
67
No longer required by the Department of Transport

1.27 DTp Special Projects
68 69 70 71

47

Vehicle Record

2.1 Record Type
1 2

[2]

1 New vehicle record
5 Amended vehicle record

2.2 Police Force
3 4

2.3 Accident Ref No
5 6 7 8 9 10 11

2.4 Vehicle Ref No
12 13 14

2.5 Type of Vehicle
15 16

01 Pedal cycle
02 Moped
03 Motor scooter
04 Motor cycle
05 Combination
06 Invalid Tricycle
07 Other three-wheeled car
08 Taxi
09 Car (four wheeled)
10 Minibus/Motor caravan
11 PSV
12 Goods not over 1 1/2 tons UW (1.52 tonnes)
13 Goods over 1 1/2 tons UW (1.52 tonnes)
14 Other motor vehicle
15 Other non motor vehicle

2.6 Towing and Articulation
17

0 No tow/articulation
1 Articulated vehicle
2 Double/multiple trailer
3 Caravan
4 Single trailer
5 Other tow

2.7 Manoeuvres
18 19

01 Reversing
02 Parked
03 Waiting to go ahead but held up
04 Stopping
05 Starting
06 U turn
07 Turning left
08 Waiting to turn left
09 Turning right
10 Waiting to turn right
11 Changing lane to left
12 Changing lane to right
13 Overtaking moving vehicle on its offside
14 Overtaking stationary vehicle on its offside
15 Overtaking on nearside
16 Going ahead left hand bend
17 Going ahead right hand bend
18 Going ahead other

2.8 Vehicle Movement Compass Point
20 21

From To

1 N   2 NE   3 E
4 SE   5 S   6 SW
7 W   8 NW

or   [0] [0] Parked - not at kerb

[0] Parked - at kerb

2.9 Vehicle Location at time of Accident
22 23

01 Leaving the main road
02 Entering the main road
03 On main road
04 On minor road
05 On service road
06 On lay-by or hard shoulder
07 Entering lay-by or hard shoulder
08 Leaving lay-by or hard shoulder
09 On a cycleway
10 Not on carriageway

2.10 Junction Location of Vehicle at First Impact
24

0 Not at junction (or within 20 metres/22 yards)
1 Vehicle approaching junction/vehicle parked at junction approach
2 Vehicle in middle of junction
3 Vehicle cleared junction/vehicle parked at junction exit
4 Did not impact

2.11 Skidding and Overturning
25

0 No skidding, jackknifing or overturning
1 Skidded
2 Skidded and overturned
3 Jackknifed
4 Jackknifed and overturned
5 Overturned

2.12 Hit Object In Carriageway
26 27

00 None
01 Previous accident
02 Road works
03 Parked vehicle - lit
04 Parked vehicle - unlit
05 Bridge (roof)
06 Bridge (side)
07 Bollard/refuge
08 Open door of vehicle
09 Central island or roundabout
10 Kerb
11 Other object

2.13 Vehicle Leaving Carriageway
28

0 Did not leave carriageway
1 Left carriageway nearside
2 Left carriageway nearside and rebounded
3 Left carriageway straight ahead at junction
4 Left carriageway offside onto central reservation
5 Left carriageway offside onto central reservation and rebounded
6 Left carriageway offside crossed central reservation
7 Left carriageway offside
8 Left carriageway offside and rebounded

2.14 Hit Object Off Carriageway
29 30

00 None
01 Road sign/Traffic signal
02 Lamp post
03 Telegraph pole/Electricity pole
04 Tree
05 Bus stop/Bus shelter
06 Central crash barrier
07 Nearside or offside crash barrier
08 Submerged in water (completely)
09 Entered ditch
10 Other permanent object

2.15 Vehicle Prefix/Suffix Letter
31

Prefix/Suffix letter or one of the following codes -

0 More than twenty years old (at end of year)
1 Unknown/cherished number/not applicable
2 Foreign/diplomatic
3 Military
4 Trade plates

2.16 First Point of Impact
32

0 Did not impact
1 Front   2 Back
3 Offside   4 Nearside

2.17 Other Vehicle Hit (VEH Ref No)
33 34 35

2.18 Part(s) Damaged
36 37 38

0 None   1 Front
2 Back   3 Offside
4 Nearside   5 Roof
6 Underside   7 all four sides

2.19 No of Axles
39

No longer required by the Department of Transport

2.20 Maximum Permissible Gross Weight
40 41

Metric tonnes (Goods vehicle only)

2.21 Sex of Driver
42

1 Male   2 Female
3 Not traced

2.22 Age of Driver
43 44

(Years estimated if necessary)

2.23 Breath Test
45

0 Not applicable   1 Positive
2 Negative   3 Not requested
4 Failed to provide
5 Driver not contacted at time

2.24 Hit and Run
46

0 Other   1 'Hit and run'
2 Non-stop vehicle not hit

2.25 DTp Special Projects
47 48 49 50

Casualty Record

3.1 Record Type
```
1 2
[3]
```
1 New casualty record
5 Amended casualty record

3.2 Police Force
```
3 4
[  ]
```

3.3 Accident Ref No
```
5 6 7 8 9 10 11
[             ]
```

3.4 Vehicle Ref No
```
12 13 14
[      ]
```

3.5 Casualty Ref No
```
15 16 17
[      ]
```

3.6 Casualty Class
```
18
[  ]
```
1 Driver or Rider
2 Vehicle or pillion passenger
3 Pedestrian

3.7 Sex of Casualty
```
19
[  ]
```
1 Male
2 Female

3.8 Age of Casualty
```
20 21
[    ]
```
(Years estimated if necessary)

3.9 Severity of Casualty
```
22
[  ]
```
1 Fatal
2 Serious
3 Slight

3.10 Pedestrian Location
```
23 24
[    ]
```
00 Not pedestrian
01 In carriageway crossing on pedestrian crossing
02 In carriageway crossing within zig-zag lines approach to the crossing
03 In carriageway crossing within zig-zag lines exit the crossing
04 In carriageway crossing elsewhere within 50 metres of pedestrian crossing
05 In carriageway crossing elsewhere
06 On footway or verge
07 On refuge or central island or reservation
08 In centre of carriageway not on refuge or central island
09 In carriageway not crossing
10 Unknown

3.11 Pedestrian Movement
```
25
[  ]
```
0 Not pedestrian
1 Crossing from drivers nearside
2 Crossing from drivers nearside - masked by parked or stationary vehicle
3 Crossing from drivers offside
4 Crossing from drivers offside - masked by parked or stationary vehicle
5 In carriageway stationary - not crossing (standing or playing)
6 In carriageway stationary - not crossing (standing or playing) - masked by parked or stationary vehicle
7 Walking along in carriageway facing traffic
8 Walking along in carriageway back to traffic
9 Unknown

3.12 Pedestrian Direction
```
26
[  ]
```
Compass point bound
1 N
2 NE
3 E
4 SE
5 S
6 SW
7 W
8 NW
or 0 - Pedestrian - standing still

3.13 School Pupil Casualty
```
27
[  ]
```
0 Not a school pupil
1 Pupil on journey to/from school
2 Pupil NOT on journey to/from school

3.14 Seat Belt Usage
```
28
[  ]
```
0 Not car or van
1 Safety belt in use
2 Safety belt fitted - not in use
3 Safety belt not fitted
4 Child safety belt/harness fitted - in use
5 Child safety belt/harness fitted - not in use
6 Child safety belt/harness not fitted
7 Unknown

3.15 Car Passenger
```
29
[  ]
```
0 Not a car passenger
1 Front seat car passenger
2 Rear seat car passenger

3.16 PSV Passenger
```
30
[  ]
```
0 Not a PSV passenger
1 Boarding
2 Alighting
3 Standing passenger
4 Seated passenger

3.17 DTp Special Projects
```
31 32 33 34
[        ]
```

Printed in the United Kingdom for HMSO
Dd 297084 C6 10/93 17434